SHATTERED LIVES:

100 VICTIMS OF GOVERNMENT HEALTH CARE

By

Amy Ridenour and Ryan Balis

THE NATIONAL CENTER
★★★
FOR PUBLIC POLICY RESEARCH

The National Center for Public Policy Research
501 Capitol Court, N.E., Suite 200, Washington, D.C. 20002
phone: (202) 543-4110, fax: (202) 543-5975
Internet: http://www.nationalcenter.org
e-mail: info@nationalcenter.org

Library of Congress Cataloging-in-Publication Data

Ridenour, Amy.
Shattered lives : 100 victims of government health care / Amy Ridenour and
Ryan Balis.
                      p. ; cm.
              ISBN 978-0-9665961-0-6
1. National health services. 2. Health care reform 3. Health services
accessibility. I. Balis, Ryan. II. National Center for Public Policy Research.
III. Title.
[DNLM: 1. State Medicine. 2. Government Regulation. 3. Health Care
Reform. 4. Health Services Accessibility. 5. Universal Coverage. W 225.1
R544s 2009]
RA412.R53 2009
362.1'0425--dc22
                                                                    2009027068

ACKNOWLEDGMENTS

The authors wish to express their thanks to the following organizations and individuals who provided valuable information or assistance.

Lauren Bean, Jack Bloom, MPL, Tom Blumer, Congressman Michael C. Burgess, M.D., *Castanet* (Kelowna, Canada), David R. Henderson, Cerere Kihoro, Mark R. Levin, Paul Mirengoff, On The Fence Films, Congressman Ron Paul, M.D., Vicky Ringer and Val Ringer of Levi's Star, *Salisbury Journal* (Salisbury, UK), Richard Sementa, Biljana Silke, Norman Singleton, Victoria Strokova and Mark Valenti's Liberty Page.

A special thanks is due to David A. Ridenour and Stephen Saunders for developing the resources to make this book possible, and to David Ridenour for contributing the title of this book and for his assistance during every stage of production. A further special acknowledgement is due to Deroy Murdock, who first conceived the idea of collecting the stories of victims of government-run health care into a book.

An extra special thanks is offered to the approximately 100,000 individual supporters of The National Center for Public Policy Research, without whose concern for our nation and generosity of spirit this book would not have been possible.

To all these individuals, we offer our grateful appreciation.

TABLE OF CONTENTS

CANADA

AUSTRALIA

INTRODUCTION

"I'll be honest; there are countries where a single-payer system works pretty well," assured President Barack Obama in a speech before the American Medical Association. The 100 worldwide victims of government-managed health care featured in this book would take issue with the President.

The reality is that wherever experiments in socialized medicine exist, the same misery follows: long wait-lists for lifesaving treatment, unequal access to health services – particularly, advanced medical technology – and an overall lack of choice in making one's own health decisions.

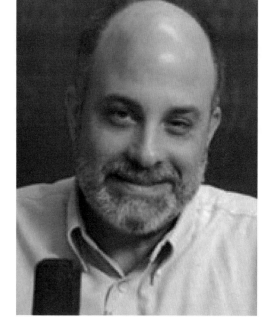

In Britain, the Department of Health considered it a welcomed improvement that the number of people on hospital waiting lists dipped below 800,000 in 2005. The shortage of doctors is so extreme in Canada that some doctors have held lotteries to reduce their caseload; the lucky "winners" lose their family doctor.

While a so-called universal health care system sounds compassionate to some, the fact is millions of citizens in these systems needlessly suffer. The reason is simple: politicians and government bureaucrats decide whether you receive treatment – not you, and not your doctor.

Take, for example, Canadian Lindsay McCreith, who had to travel across the border to a Buffalo hospital when he was told it would take over four months to get a scan of his brain tumor and a further eight months to remove it in Canada. As an editorial in Canada's National Post put it, had he put his full faith and trust in the Canadian government health system, "Lindsay McCreith would likely be dead today."

Universal systems are promoted as 'free care!' Who among us isn't tempted by more of something paid for by someone else? But, of course, in these socialist so-called Meccas, government health programs cannot escape basic economics.

The immense cost of providing taxpayer-funded health care has forced countries with a nationalized system to place severe limits on the supply of health services. They do this by putting patients on long waiting lists or by denying them effective medications outright, thereby rationing care. Patients wait sometimes years for vital treatment and often do not receive the newest and best drugs.

When you wait, you wait in pain and sometimes die.

While health care reform is all the rage in Washington these days, many of our elected leaders in Washington are looking in all the wrong places. A big government solution as envisioned by politicians such as President Obama and Nancy Pelosi would forever limit Americans' access to life-saving treatment and would massively increase the size and scope of government's involvement in the economy — and in our private medical decisions.

Does America's health care system have its problems? You bet. But improving health care should involve giving people more power to control their own health decisions.

My hope is that *Shattered Lives* will educate you, the American public, to the horror of government-managed health care where it exists today.

In this book are documented stories from Canada, the United Kingdom, South Africa, Japan, Australia and elsewhere – countries in which citizens literally die waiting for health services. Among other horrifying takes, you will cringe over tales of expectant mothers unable to find an available hospital bed, elderly patients denied routine cataract surgery and people in agony who resorted to do-it-yourself dentistry.

These tragic stories warn us that turning more of our health care decisions over to the government is sure to bring us nothing but pain.

Mark R. Levin
Host, *The Mark Levin Show*
Author, *Liberty and Tyranny: A Conservative Manifesto*

PREFACE

There's no such thing as a free lunch, but the government keeps trying to sell us one anyway.

And so it is with government-run health care. Sold to the public in the guise of "free," it is in fact more costly than any private alternative, for its price tag is more than financial. Those who chose to rely on government health care frequently pay not just in taxes, but in a more costly currency: pain, fear, suffering and death.

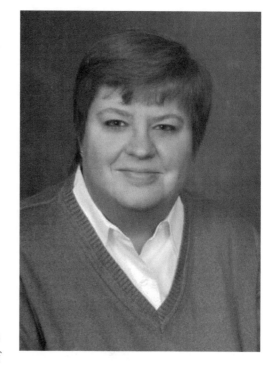

In the pages that follow you will find 100 stories telling the tales of people who paid a costly price within their nation's government-run health care system. They come from all walks of life. Some are poor, some are working or middle class and some are at the highest echelons of their societies. One, at the time his story took place, was a prime minister.

In some of these tales, the difficulties encountered are relatively minor – a person spending a few days without any food, for example. In others, the story ends in death.

Had we chosen to do so, we could have filled this entire book exclusively with stories of people who died because the public health system in their country is structurally unable to meet the vital health care needs of its citizenry. It has been estimated, for example, that in Britain alone 25,000 people die every year from cancer whose lives could have been saved or meaningfully extended[1] had they had access to drugs and treatments Americans mostly take for granted. We do have several of those stories in this book. But as the failure of government-run medicine is so much more pervasive than its administators' common refusal to prescribe expensive but lifesaving cancer drugs, we have endeavored instead to paint a much fuller picture.

As we tell these stories, it may be helpful for the reader to know a bit about the health systems in the various nations we cover. To follow, then, is a quick snapshot for each:

Great Britain: Britain has a single-payer government-run system financed by taxes and administered by local Primary Care Trusts, which directly employ doctors, nurses, midwives and other medical personnel. Private medical and dental services also exist and are legal, as is private health insurance. Approximately 10 percent of Britons have some form of private health insurance.

Canada: Canada has a single-payer government-run system financed by taxes and administered at the provincial level. Canadians have been discouraged, and in some cases, banned, from privately supplying or acquiring those medical services offered by the public system, although these bans been under legal challenge in recent years.

Australia: Australia has a universal care system in which a public system paid for by tax revenue co-exists with a much smaller private system. The public system covers the full cost of public hospital stays and doctor visits, and subsidizes other good and services, including prescription drugs.

South Africa: South Africa has a public system financed by tax dollars and used by approximately 80 percent of the population. Services are free to pregnant women and children under six; other patients pay a fee for services based on their ability to pay. A private system with substantially higher quality of care co-exists with the public one.

Japan: Japan has a complicated universal system funded by mandatory payroll and other taxes based largely on place and type of employment and age. The government sets the price of all medical services, and residents make co-payments for medical services that are roughly 10-30 percent of the government-determined price of those services.

Russia: Russia has a public system that officially is free for all, but in which corruption – in which medical service providers require bribes before providing services – is a severe problem. A private health market is legal and a small portion of the citizenry carries private health insurance.

Sweden: Sweden has a publicly-financed universal system largely administered by elected local councils, which have tax-levying powers, although the national government sets general policy, supervises the activities of the councils and contributes some financing from national tax revenue. Private health care is legal in Sweden but heavily regulated. In the 1990s, some limited market reforms were introduced in an effort to reduce waiting lists.

New Zealand: New Zealand's system is similar to Britain's, in which a large public system available to all and financed by general taxation co-exists with a much smaller private system, with private health insurance legal. In the public system, no payment is required for hospital stays, for emergency treatment, for most diagnostic tests, for treatment by specialists, along with certain other services. Prescription drugs are subsidized.

While absorbing these stories, the reader may desire a fuller picture of some of the health care challenges facing residents of the countries we've covered. The following statistics provide a glimpse of that fuller picture:

In Britain in 2007, only 47 percent of cancer patients requiring postoperative radiotherapy received it within the government's "maximum acceptable delay" of four weeks.[2] Some post-operative patients saw cancer return before radiation began.[3]

In Britain in 2006, 53,181 surgeries were cancelled at the last minute due to shortages or errors, while approximately 250,000 surgeries, about 962 per day, were cancelled altogether in England that year.[4]

At the end of 2006, 775,468 Britons were on waiting lists to be admitted to a hospital for treatment. 185,527 had been waiting three to six months.[5]

Based solely on cost, Britain's National Health Service has for years denied the four best available drugs to kidney cancer patients in Britain, leaving as many with the choice only of Interferon, to which as many as three-quarters do not meaningfully respond,[6] or essentially being left to die. In 2007, the Times quoted a Birmingham oncologist saying of Nexavar: "Patients with this cancer tend to die quite quickly but I know from my own patients who were on the trial how well this drug works. They are still alive two years later."[7] In February 2009, after years of pleas by physicians and kidney cancer patients and their advocates, Britain's National Institute for Health and Clinical Excellence (NICE) finally relented in the case of one of the drugs, Sutent, but continued to block NHS use of Nexavar, Avastin and Torisel to treat this cancer,[8] although they are in wide use for this purpose in the U.S. and much of Europe.

Patients with rare cancers in Britain have been denied potentially lifesaving drugs because their cancers are too rare to have received attention from NICE, the NHS's drug approval board. Because NHS doctors are forbidden to prescribe drugs outside NICE's specifications, patients with these cancers are forced to beg for NHS coverage on a case-by-case basis, and often are rejected.[9]

Though Britons routinely are denied potentially-lifesaving cancer drugs because of their cost, the same health service funds "shaman therapies," through which patients supposedly can receive "soul retrieval healing" to help the "continue their journey into the hereafter" and investigate "the Fairy Kingdom."[10] Other services paid for by the NHS include breast reduction and enlargements, nose jobs, liposuction, laser hair removal, tattoo removal, impotence drugs,[11] contraceptives and abortions,[12] and sex-change operations.[13]

The cancer death rate is 70 percent higher in the United Kingdom than in the U.S.[14]

The British National Health Service typically limits what it will pay to extend a life by six months to $22,000.[15]

In Canada in 2006, the average wait after a referral to a specialist until treatment was 17.8 weeks. Canadians waited 10.3 weeks for MRIs and 4.3 weeks for CT scans, on average.[16] In Saskatchewan, 42 percent of patients needing orthopedic surgery had to wait four months or more; 14 percent had to wait over a year.[17]

Over 1,500 ear, nose and throat surgery patients in Australia have waited over eight years for surgery. Experts say some will never get it, because more urgent surgery cases will always be put above them in waiting lines.[18]

Twice as many Canadians as Americans report waiting more than four hours to be seen in an emergency room, said the Canadian Fraser Institute in 2006.[19]

Overcrowding in Canadian hospitals is so bad that some patients are forced to sleep in closets and nurse's lounges.[20]

A February 2007 survey by the Canadian Spine Society found that some patients with debilitating and painful back problems were on waiting lists for up to six years for treatment. Some back specialists had over 1,000 patients waiting for appointments.[21]

New Zealanders and Australians were more than twice as likely, Canadians four times as likely, and Britons five times as likely to be forced to wait four months or more for elective surgery as were Americans, according to Canada's Fraser Institute in 2006. Americans were twice as likely as Canadians, Britons, New Zealanders or Australians to believe they could get an appointment to see a specialist within one week.[22]

19% of Americans with prostate cancer die from it, while 25% of Canadians, 30% of New Zealanders, 35% of Australians and 57% of Britons who have it die from it.[23]

25% of Americans with breast cancer die from it, while 28% of Canadians, 28% of Australians, 46% of New Zealanders and 46% of Britons with breast cancer die from it.[24]

A doctor at a public hospital in South Africa revealed in March 2007 that the waiting list at his hospital for hernia repair is three years, and for hip and knee surgeries, 18 years.[25]

American politicians have of late been extremely critical of the American health care system, and there are constructive criticisms that can be made. No one denies the U.S. system has room for improvement. But as we consider the statistics above, and the plight of individuals in the stories that follow, it becomes clear that we Americans have a great deal about which to be grateful.

Amy Ridenour
President
The National Center for Public Policy Research

ENGINEER LEFT BLIND FOR THREE YEARS AWAITING 20-MINUTE OPERATION

According to Britain's state-managed health service, cataract surgery is a "common" and "straightforward" operation that usually should last between 15 and 20 minutes.[1] But such a quick turnaround would have been news to Richard Adams of London, who went blind in both eyes while waiting three years for cataract surgery.

The 85-year-old retired engineer and award-winning dancer began losing his vision in 2004. That year, doctors diagnosed Adams with cataracts, but an operation to remove them was not scheduled until March 2007.[2]

His excitement in 2007 at the prospect of getting his sight and livelihood back was short-lived because doctors cancelled the surgery.

"I was over the moon when I found out I had an appointment in March [2007] but when it was cancelled I just went downhill," Adams said at the time.[3]

Stuck in a wheelchair and suffering from asthma as well as kidney stones (also left untreated by the NHS, he said), Adams had difficulty performing everyday tasks. "I never cook anything," Adams explained then. "It always has to be cold things like sandwiches or salad. I can't go to the shops because I can't see where I'm going."[4]

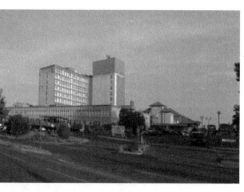

Ealing Hospital was one of several hospitals that refused to provide cataract surgery for 85-year-old Richard Adams, who went blind as a result.

In despair, Adams said his life was "being wasted": "I have all these ideas in my head but I can't see to write and I can't see to draw. All I can do is sit in my house and listen to the TV. I can't see it and I have to turn up the volume because I can't hear well."[5]

Spokesman Mark Purcell of Ealing Hospital, one of several hospitals that refused Adams treatment for his eyes, offered no sympathy. "If [Adams] has a complaint about the standard of care he has received he should write to the chief executive of the Ealing Hospital Trust."[6] (Whether this bureaucratic solution, which asked a blind man to write, was intentionally or inadvertently cruel is unknown.)

Adams was scheduled to receive treatment in late May, but this was little consolation for him. "I've been waiting for three years but they don't seem to care. I think they're just waiting for me to die or something," Adams complained.[8]

Finally, after Adams' plight received attention from the British press, doctors removed the cataracts in one of his eyes in June 2007.[8]

"He was really pleased with the result of the operation," said Roger Woolsey, a family friend. "When I went to visit him he would raise the eye-patch and say: I really can see again."[9]

Tragically, four days after the procedure that restored his sight, Adams died. He had a heart attack after developing blood poisoning in the hospital.[10]

NHS NIGHTMARE: REPEATED SURGERY CANCELLATIONS KILL ELDERLY CANCER PATIENT

Mavis Skeet, 74, of West Yorkshire, United Kingdom was diagnosed with cancer of the esophagus,[11] an aggressive throat cancer that kills 90 percent of victims within five years of diagnosis.[12]

In early December 1999, following a scan showing that the cancer had not spread,[13] doctors were due to remove Skeet's gullet and to surgically determine the extent of the disease.[14] Skeet's family had hoped the growth would be treated in time for Christmas.[15]

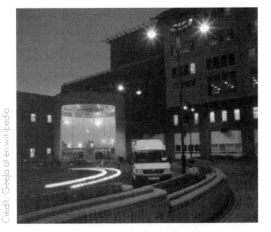
Credit: Geejo at en.wikipedia

Mavis Skeet desperately needed surgery before her cancer spread, but after her surgery was cancelled four times – three times because the hospital lacked intensive care beds – it became inoperable.

However, the operation scheduled that December at Leeds General Infirmary was cancelled because one of the members of the surgery team, an anesthesiologist, had the flu.[16] As the winter flu season progressed over the coming weeks, Skeet's surgery was cancelled another three times because the hospital lacked available intensive care beds.[17]

Dr. Hugo Mascie-Taylor, medical director for the Leeds hospital, reasoned, "It would have been irresponsible to have carried out the operation when we could not have been sure of having an intensive care bed available."[18] But on one occasion, surgery was cancelled as Skeet was being moved to the operating room "because her intensive care bed was needed by another patient," according to a BBC report.[19]

"It's heartbreaking. The whole point of her going into hospital was to have an emergency operation," said daughter Jane Skeet.[20] "We are very angry. The doctors say they can't tell whether the cancer's spread until they operate, which means it could be spreading all the time while there's a lack of beds."[21]

Unfortunately, Jane Skeet's fears were realized. As the cancer progressed, Mavis Skeet had to be fed through an intravenous drip because the tumor prevented her from swallowing.[22] By the time doctors got around to work on Skeet in January 2000 – five weeks after the initial scheduled operation – it was too late. The cancer had spread to her windpipe in two places, and doctors determined the tumor was inoperable.[23]

"I know that if she'd had the operation five weeks ago the cancer would not have spread to her windpipe," said an angry Jane Skeet.[24] "Had they operated five weeks ago the tumor was operable and could have been removed. Now they can't operate."[25]

For five months, Jane helplessly watched her mother's condition deteriorate, until Mavis Skeet passed away in late May 2000.[26] Jane puts blame for her mother's death squarely on the British National Health Service. "This is due to lack of resources and bad planning," she said. "The government is trying to cover it up by saying the hospitals are coping, but they're obviously not."[27]

In frustration, Jane wrote to then-Prime Minister Tony Blair, detailing her mother's astounding experience with the NHS: "How can you justify the loss of a life because of the lack of a suitable bed? ...We placed our mother's life in the hands of your Health Service and it has killed her. My mother is a devout Christian and she had helped her church raise funds for hospitals. It is a cruel irony that this is how she is repaid.

"I look at my mother and I still can't believe she is going to die, but we know she will. She will because the NHS let her down in the most crucial five weeks of her entire life."[28]

EX-BRITISH MP AND LONGTIME NATIONAL HEALTH SERVICE SUPPORTER DENIED SIGHT-SAVING DRUG

To save an arm, a leg or even an eye, would you rethink deeply held principles?

12 Great Britain

This was the dilemma that faced the decidedly left-wing former Member of Parliament,[29] Alice Mahon. Mahon was going blind because of a decision by the government-managed National Health Service, which she had long supported as a member of the Labour Party,[30] Britain's traditionally left party that launched the NHS in 1948.[31]

Mahon suffers from the 'wet' type of age-related macular degeneration (ARMD). The condition requires early treatment because it progresses rapidly, resulting in severely impaired vision and possibly blindness.[32] Mahon thought she was fortunate because doctors in November 2006 prescribed to her a newly-available drug in the

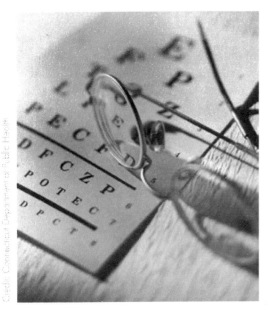

United Kingdom, Lucentis, to treat her eyes. Clinical trials showed the drug to be effective at stabilizing vision loss and even reversing damage.[33]

But, unhappily for Mahon, at that time government funding for Lucentis had not been approved. In hopes of speeding up the process, Mahon sent an urgent application to an "exceptional circumstances" review committee through her local health authority, Calderdale and Kirklees Primary Care Trust. But it took nine weeks from the original application date for the committee to turn down funding Mahon's prescription whose cost would be 12,000 British pounds (~$19,500) for a year's treatment.[34]

No Member of Parliament was a bigger fan of the government health system than Alice Mahon – until the system, to save money, decided to let her go blind.

As Mahon explained, "I was given two reasons for the refusal – firstly, the treatment I need has not been approved by NICE [National Institute for Health and Clinical Excellence – the clinical standards body], and secondly, it has not been proven to be effective. Neither reason stands up to scrutiny."[35]

Meanwhile, during the lengthy review process, Mahon lost much of her sight in one eye. Fearing irreversible vision loss, she began treatment on her own, that is, with her own money.[36] Though Mahon and her husband could afford to pay for treatment using their retirement savings,[37] the thought of buying private health care was outlandish to her.

"It went against every principle of mine to consider private health care," said Mahon.[38] "Everyone has a right to free treatment on the NHS for a condition that results in blindness and devastates lives."[39]

Mahon continued, "[M]y husband Tony was all for me going private... but I refused... I'd been a [Labour] party member since 1957. My grandfather was a founder member. This was my NHS: I had been its champion all my life and it would not let me down. How I regret that proud stance now."[40]

Yet, having few viable options to save her vision, Mahon purchased private care. By the end of January 2007, she had spent £5,325 (~$8,700) on treatment.[41] Says a distressed Mahon, "I have been an ardent supporter of the NHS all my life, and now feel totally let down. The excuses... for not funding treatment are scandalously lame."[42]

Mahon contemplated suing the NHS, but she did not proceed because, finally, health officials agreed to pay for Lucentis. Yet it appeared other, less politically-connected sufferers of ARMD were not as fortunate as Mahon. According to policy, to receive Lucentis through the NHS, patients must already have been blind in one eye and show deterioration in the other eye.[43]

NICE reversed this policy in 2008 to permit NHS funding for the first 14 injections of Lucentis as soon as wet age-related macular degeneration is diagnosed in one eye. The drug's manufacturer, Novartis, will pay for any additional doses under the new guidelines. According to the Daily Mail, it is believed that some 20,000 patients lost their sight during the two-year review considering new guidelines.[44]

DEATH BY BUREAUCRACY IN BRITAIN'S GOVERNMENT HEALTH SERVICE

Imagine losing a loved one, only to be offered a "remedy" one year later.

Pat Booy of Bristol, United Kingdom lost her husband, Brian, 60, to a heart attack. Brian had been on the government-managed Bristol Royal Infirmary's waiting list for triple heart bypass surgery for 72 weeks since doctors diagnosed him with angina in July 1997.[45]

Not wanting to risk missing Brian's surgery, the family took great lengths to stay by his side. "We were frightened to go out or go on holiday in case the phone rang and we missed it. He was looking forward to the life he was going to lead after the operation," said Pat.[46]

But Brian's turn never came. After being taken to Southmead Hospital because of breathing difficulties in January 1999, Brian was diagnosed with a chest infection. Two days later, a massive heart attack killed Brian at home.[47]

Says a frustrated Pat, "When they told us we were on the waiting list we just accepted it, thinking it might be a few months. But it just went on and on and in the end you just think it will never happen. Angina is not the sort of thing you can wait for. It just gets worse and it needs to be dealt with straight away."[48]

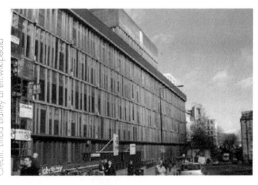

Credit: Linda Bailey at en.wikipedia

Brian Booy spent 72 weeks on the triple heart bypass surgery waiting list of the Bristol Royal Infirmary (pictured) before dying of a massive heart attack. A year after his death, his family was told Brian could have the surgery in two months.

"I can't believe it could ever have got that bad without something being done," Pat added.[49]

However, at roughly the time of the one-year mark of Brian's death, widow Pat received a letter from the cardiac department at Bristol Royal Infirmary. Finally, Brian was offered an appointment for heart bypass surgery for the beginning of March 2000 – over one year since his death. A baffled and angry Pat said, "It was a bit of an angry scene. I thought 'Surely they must know' [of Brian's death], and my son was very angry and phoned the hospital."[50]

Astonishingly, the hospital had not recorded Brian's death. A hospital spokesman explained, "At present the hospital does not have a way of knowing if a patient has died unless we are informed by a GP [general practitioner – *i.e.*, family doctor]."[51]

Two years after Brian's death, a frustrated Pat remarked, "I know what it is like to live your life on a waiting list and it's no fun. When you are dealing with someone's heart, there is no such thing as a non-urgent case. I don't want anyone else to go through what we have."[52]

"I can't help but wonder," Brian's widow added, "that if he'd had the operation sooner, he'd still be here."[53]

DO-IT-YOURSELF DENTISTRY IN BRITAIN

"I was lying awake at night being driven mad by this constant throbbing ache; it was horrible," recalls George Daulat of Scarborough, England.[54] Over the course of several weeks, Daulat had developed a nasty toothache.[55] When the pain became unbearable, Daulat's girlfriend helped him look for treatment. She made calls to 20 public National Health Service dentists as well as private practices, though Daulat was unemployed.[56]

However, because of a shortage of dentists, there was no dentist available. In fact, Scarborough residents needed to travel over 50 miles to other towns just to receive a check up or filling.[57] The British The Sun newspaper reported in 2004 that Scarborough:

> [I]s so hard-hit with the lack of NHS dentists that queues stretched hundreds of yards earlier this year [February 2004] when one finally opened... Around 3,000 people tried to join [register for care] – but they were left stranded when Dutch dentist Aria Van Drie fled after it was revealed she had criminal convictions.[58]

In desperation, Daulat decided to do the work the old fashioned way – by himself, using old rusty pliers.

"I knew it would hurt but I thought 'just suffer it' rather than go through extended pain," Daulat said.[59] "In the end I simply could take any more."[60] He added: "I had a pair of pliers in a tool box. They were old and a bit rusty but I knew they would do the job."[61]

Daulat bought a bottle of vodka as anesthetic and to dull the pain, and drank a pint of it before pulling the first ailing tooth. Daulat describes the gruesome process in detail:

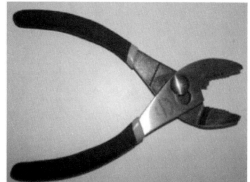

> I gripped the first tooth, squeezed and pulled. I felt this blinding pain, followed by a snap as the tooth cracked... I pulled again and managed to get the whole thing out... However, the pain was still there and I went back for two more. I managed to get them out but the fourth wouldn't come... I tugged and tugged but I couldn't get it out and I have had to leave it halfway out.[62]

George Doulat's dentistry instrument of choice after 20 public NHS dentist offices were too busy to remove his four bad teeth (model shown).

In agony, Daulat called the local NHS emergency dentist center, Northway Clinic, for immediate care. But Northway refused to see Daulat the day he pulled the teeth because his call was not made early enough in the day.[63]

At last, the next day Daulat was treated at a local NHS dentistry after the practice read about Daulat's handling in the newspaper.

"He was obviously in agony and we wanted to help him," said Kasandra Dowling of Medimatch dental practice in Scarborough. Though relieved, Daulat said: "I'm so happy I've got a dentist and I'm not in pain anymore but did it really have to go this far before somebody did something?"[65]

He added, "People will think I am crazy to have pulled my own teeth out but they weren't living with the pain."[66] "It was the hardest and most horrible thing I have ever done, but I was desperate."[67]

NATIONAL HEALTH SERVICE DENIED SIGHT-SAVING MEDICINE TO ITS OWN EMPLOYEE

An employee of Britain's government-run National Health Service was denied medication that could save her from going blind in one eye.

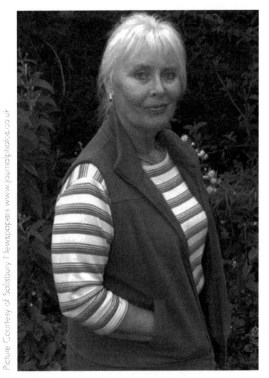

Picture Courtesy of Salisbury Newspapers www.journalphotos.co.uk

After 18 years of service to the NHS, Sylvie Webb fought her employer for nearly a year when it denied her the drugs she needed to save her sight.

Sylvie Webb, a widow from Salisbury, England, worked for 18 years as a secretary at Salisbury District Hospital.[68] Yet, despite her situation, Webb discovered that medical treatment under the public health service is anything but universal.

In February 2007, doctors diagnosed Webb, then 58, with the "wet" type of age-related macular degeneration (ARMD) in her left eye.[69] If not treated in a timely manner, wet ARMD "can lead to blindness in as little as three months and people need prompt treatment if they are to minimize the risk of permanent sight loss," according to a statement by the Royal National Institute of Blind People in London.[70]

As such, Webb's medical consultant sought rapid treatment for Webb because her sight was "deteriorating 'day by day,'" as Webb explained,[71] and an infection in one eye can spread to the other good eye.[72]

But to Webb's dismay, for nearly a year her local public health authority, Dorset Primary Care Trusts, refused to provide Webb with the expensive "anti-VEGF" drugs she desperately needed to save her sight.[72] Though two such effective drugs, Macugen and Lucentis,[73] are licensed for general NHS use, the Dorset Trust, which controls funding prescriptions, dragged its feet. Dorset Trust said it has yet to formulate a policy in a "fair and equitable way"[74] to treat Webb's condition and thus it could not provide her with the VEGF drugs.[75]

As Webb explained then, "At the time, the PCT [Dorset Primary Care Trusts] said it hadn't got a policy and it would address the situation in April [2007] – but it has now postponed this until June. I'm extremely worried that time is running out for me and other patients."[76]

The prospect of going blind terrified Webb:

> I'm a young woman and want to carry on working, and then I'd like to do all the things I had planned for my retirement. I'm also worried about the health of my other eye. I know I'm at increased risk of getting wet AMD in that eye and this could mean I end up losing my sight. The women in my family live into their 90s; I can't accept the possibility of being blind unnecessarily for the next 35 years.[77]

In May 2007, the Trust agreed to review Webb's case on an urgent basis. But for Tom Bremridge, CEO of the Macular Disease Society in Andover, UK, there is no excuse for Webb being without the available sight-saving drugs she needs. "It is outrageous that in this day and age Mrs. Webb faces losing her sight owing to bureaucratic idleness," he said.[78]

Steve Winyard of RNIB echoed Bremridge's outrage:

> This is disgraceful... It's little comfort for Mrs. Webb that she can't get treatment simply because her PCT has yet to decide a policy. The PCT needs to get its act together and ensure these drugs are available to patients now and without a struggle... There is a moral imperative to save the sight of people where we can.[79]

Finally, in 2008 new health guidelines permitted Dorset Trusts to prescribe Lucentis for Webb. The guidelines published by the National Institute for Clinical Excellence, the government's health advisory authority, allow for funding for the first 14 injections of Lucentis once wet ARMD is diagnosed in one eye. If additional injections are necessary, the drug's manufacturer, Novartis, will pay for additional treatment.[80]

Webb was delighted that she would at last receive the sight-saving drug. "I'm so relieved that Dorset PCT has finally realized the long-term benefit to me of this treatment and has agreed funding," she said. "I only hope that all patients are given treatment to help save their sight because while this is good news for me, there may be hundreds of others with wet AMD who cannot get the funding they desperately need."[81]

SOME BRITISH DOCTORS COULDN'T OFFER EXPENSIVE LIFE-SAVING CANCER DRUG

Jackie O'Donnell of Middlesbrough, England needed aggressive treatment to survive advanced ovarian cancer, which doctors had diagnosed in late 1998.[82]

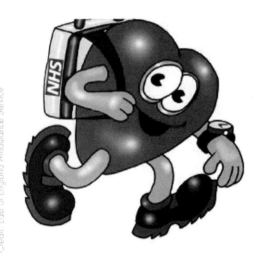

After unsuccessful surgery, O'Donnell had five inoperable tumors.[83] Yet, her oncologist recommended a platinum-based drug, not Taxol,[84] an expensive yet powerful chemotherapy drug that attacks tumors and is widely used in the U.S., Europe and even other locations in Britain.[85] If taken at the time of diagnosis, Taxol prolongs the life of cancer sufferers 14 months on average, and patients have a 50 percent chance of survival.[86]

Despite Taxol's life-saving potential, O'Donnell discovered to her amazement that her doctor was forbidden to recommend it.

As O'Donnell explained, "I phoned my consultant back and he said yes – that [Taxol] is definitely what you need. He seemed relieved. He wasn't allowed to tell me because the health authority wouldn't pay for Taxol, which costs 1,500 pounds (~$2,400) a session and you need six to eight treatments."[87]

The NHS may advertise itself as health care with a heart, but when cancer patient Jackie O'Donnell needed the one drug that could possibly save her life, the NHS refused to provide it.

Credit: East of England Ambulance Service

O'Donnell's faith in the government-managed National Health Service was shattered. "I just didn't believe it, because in this country we were brought up to believe that we would get the best treatment available," said O'Donnell.[88] She continued, "You just trust doctors, don't you? You trust the hospital to give you the best treatment available. And then something like this smacks you in the face."[89]

Nevertheless, the local health authority, South Tees, would not fund Taxol because of its expense.[91] Facing a threat to her life, O'Donnell had no choice but to receive it without the help of the public health system. "My cancer was very advanced and I just felt so angry that I was going to be denied this chance of life that I couldn't accept that," she said.[91]

Bills for Taxol's treatment piled up, and O'Donnell and her husband, Geoff, decided they would remortgage their home if need be. "I stuffed them [bills] in the drawer and tried to forget about them, because I was fighting for my life, and I knew I didn't have the money to pay. It is disgusting really and it does upset me to think that the NHS could come to this," said O'Donnell.[92]

Curiously, though the O'Donnells paid for Taxol on their own, thanks to the "postcode lottery," in which there are significant differences in access to care and treatment depending on one's postcode, or locality, it happened to be publicly available to residents nearby through the NHS.

"If I had lived just two miles away, I could have had Taxol because the health authority in North Yorkshire did pay for it," explained O'Donnell. "I really didn't believe the postcode lottery existed until it happened to me."[93]

O'Donnell summed it up: "It's where you live deciding whether you live."[94]

Outraged, O'Donnell visited the local health authority's office to demand a face-to-face meeting with its chief executive and got her Member of Parliament involved to seek change.[95] "I became quite a firebrand."[96] Because of her vocal and persistent campaign, South Tees changed its policy in April 1999 to fund Taxol for ovarian cancer sufferers.[97]

"Other women in my position backed away. I think they felt they might have been victimized. I think they thought the hospital must know best," said O'Donnell.[98] "I don't even want to contemplate what would have happened on cheaper chemotherapy. I know women who were ill at the same time who, sadly, are not doing so well."[99]

O'Donnell referred to Taxol as "a wonder drug."[100] It would extend her life more than three years.

Though O'Donnell's cancer disappeared within three months of treatment with Taxol, O'Donnell passed away in August 2002 at the age of 57.[101]

CENTENARIAN TOLD TO WAIT 18 MONTHS TO GET HEARING AID

Longevity apparently does not count for much in Britain's government-managed National Health Service.

Much of 108-year-old's Olive Beal's hearing was gone. The one-time suffragette and former piano teacher from Kent, England was unable to enjoy music or hear conversations clearly with her five-year-old analog hearing aid.[102] A modern, digital device would improve Beal's hearing — and life — tremendously, but she was having difficulty receiving a replacement.

Beal's granddaughter, Maria Scott, explained: "Her analog hearing aid does not filter out background noise so it makes it very difficult for her to hear clearly. But the digital one would allow her to hear people talking to her and to CDs. She loves music hall numbers."[103]

Beal was administered a hearing test in late July 2007, and a hearing expert recommended a digital hearing device.[104] However, the local health authority, Eastern and Coastal Kent Primary Care Trust, has an 18-month waiting list for new hearing aids provided through the NHS. Despite her age and despite contributing income taxes that fund the government's universal health system into her late 60s, Beal was told she must wait her turn in line. A spokesman for the Eastern and Coastal Kent Primary Care Trust explained: "[P]riority is given to patients who do not have an existing hearing aid..."[105]

Under the government system, Beal would be 110 years old by the time the new hearing aid was scheduled to arrive.[106]

Beal expressed her fear: "I could be dead by then."[107]

Maria Scott added, "I would have thought they would take her age into account as she probably has not got 18 months to wait... Her eyesight is falling [sic], and if she cannot hear then she will be isolated from the outside world."[108]

Fortunately, widespread press attention and concern about Beal's situation prompted Phillip Ball, a private audiologist, to assist Beal voluntarily. Ball said:

> I can see no reason why a lady of her age should be fobbed off by her NHS Trust and told to wait at least 18 months, so I immediately got on the phone

to offer my services. I visited Olive this week and she should have a fully functioning digital aid in a matter of days [early August 2007]. She will now be able to hear a great deal better.[110]

A digital hearing device costs approximately 1,000 British pounds (~$1,600) each,[110] and wait times for hearing aids can be over two years in some parts of Britain.[111]

"The new digital hearing aids can really transform people's lives," said Donna Tipping of the Royal National Institute for the Deaf, a British charity. "It is an issue of quality of life, with isolation, frustration and withdrawing from society caused by loss of hearing, and it is sad because this is reversible."[112]

As her grandmother is one of Britain's oldest living citizens,[113] Maria Scott added, "I thought a 108-year-old deserved to be treated better than this."[114]

EIGHT HOSPITAL VISITS LATER, SIX-YEAR-OLD DIES OF LONG-UNDETECTED BRAIN TUMOR

Vicky Ringer knew something was seriously wrong with the health of her six-year-old son, Levi.

Though Levi had experienced eating and dietary problems since birth, beginning in December 2005, his health appeared to be worsening. After he complained of intense headaches and suffering dizzy spells, Levi was taken to Pinderfields Hospital in Wakefield, England in January 2006 to be examined.[115]

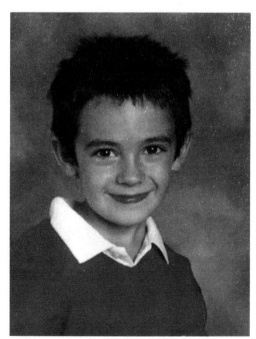

Levi was prescribed medication by a doctor who thought the headaches were caused by "eating problems and constipation."[116] But the medicine did not stop the headaches, and Vicky became increasingly worried. She took Levi back to the hospital in March, but again he was released the following day and prescribed migraine tablets.[117]

"I didn't even ask for a brain scan because I didn't know at that point that it was procedure at all," recalled

Delays in ordering a brain scan for young Levi Ringer cost him his life.

Vicky. "I would have asked if I had known, but they just sent him home and said it was a bad headache. You just listen to what you are told because they are the experts, not you."[118]

Levi's awful headaches continued into April. He also was awakening at night, sick, losing weight and becoming withdrawn. Vicky took Levi to a pediatrician, Dr. Steve Jones, as well as to a dietician, who suggested that a psychiatrist examine Levi for "behavioral problems."[119] Unsatisfied and frustrated that there was not a firm diagnosis for the cause of Levi's headaches, Vicky demanded additional tests.

"I pushed every step of the way to try and get a diagnosis, not just to keep giving him more migraine medication," she said.[120] "At that stage I was desperate to find out what was wrong with him."[121]

Yet, Vicky was still unable to convince doctors to treat Levi's case seriously and perform a brain scan. She explained:

> As his mum, I knew he wasn't well. But I was made to feel neurotic. I asked whether it could have been a brain tumor, but they disregarded it because Levi wasn't displaying what doctors call the usual symptoms. I knew in my heart it was something more serious and I persistently kept taking him back.[122]

Meanwhile, Levi's condition deteriorated. "It got to the point where he was getting headaches every day," said Vicky. "He started with dizzy spells and was too scared to lie down. He was losing weight and being sick but still there was no mention of a scan until I pushed for it."[123]

At last, Vicky's determination paid off when she convinced doctors to bypass the three-month waiting list to perform a brain scan. On July 20, seven months after the Ringers first visited a hospital and during their sixth visit overall, a scan revealed a "lollipop-size" cancerous brain tumor.[124] A supplemental scan at Leeds General Infirmary showed the cancer had, unfortunately, already spread to the boy's spine.[125]

The following day doctors performed an emergency operation to remove the tumor, but Levi would never recover.[126] Five weeks after the operation was performed (on his eighth hospital visit), Levi died of respiratory failure after life support was removed.[127]

"I said to him, 'It's ok, you can go now baby.' I didn't want him to suffer any more," recalled Vicky.[128]

"My heart is broken," said Vicky. "I put my trust in the doctors to save my son and I feel incredibly let down and angry that they didn't listen to me."[129] She added, "[If] they had noticed his symptoms and recognized what was wrong earlier – just given him the scan no matter what the cost to the NHS – he may be still alive today."[130]

Following Levi's death, Vicky pursued a negligence case against Pinderfields Hospital, arguing that the doctors had a duty to diagnose Levi's tumor earlier. "It is important to raise awareness of the signs of brain tumours in young people and fight for the rights of parents' concerns to be taken seriously." said Vicky.[131] Ultimately, the lawsuit was unsuccessful, despite an internal investigation that criticized the hospital.[132]

Vicky and Levi's grandmother, Val Ringer, formed Levi's Star, a charity to support children with brain tumors and their families. In April 2009, 100 people in Newmillerdam, England gathered for a charity walk in Levi's memory and to raise funds for Levi's Star. "I find it very respectful that people are still remembering Levi almost three years on," said Vicky.[133]

SMALL BOY TOLD TO WAIT SIX MONTHS TO GET PAINFUL TEETH REMOVED

Five-year-old Finn McEwan-Paterson of Wilmslow, England had two painful teeth. Nevertheless, the youngster's mother, Karen Walker, was told that, because of an area-wide shortage of specialist dentists, it would be six months before the offending teeth could be pulled.[134]

In late January 2006, Finn was taken to the White Dental Spa surgery for examination. The consultation revealed both teeth needed to be extracted by a specialist, with the procedure to take place at the Weston Clinic, in the nearby town of Macclesfield.[135] But three weeks after the referral was made, Karen received a letter saying there would be a six-month wait for an appointment. Unable to follow up with the clinic by phone, Karen returned in person to ask for an urgent substitute referral to a dental center in Manchester.[136]

Without finding any luck, Karen brought Finn unannounced to the Weston Clinic, the original referral clinic. Karen hoped to persuade the staff there to take pity on Finn, but she was told Finn would have to wait for an appointment. Karen and Finn were also turned away at the Manchester Dental Hospital accident and emergency department because they did not have a referral letter.[137]

"He is a five-year-old-boy who everyone acknowledges is in pain and needs his tooth taken out," said Karen. "I'm astonished that in this day and age there is nothing that can be done to relieve his pain. All he needs is his tooth out."[138]

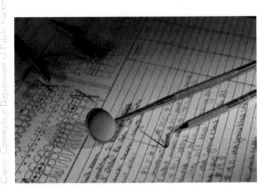

Five-year-old Finn McEwan-Paterson's teeth were so bad, his face swelled up like a chipmunk's. The waiting list to get the teeth pulled was six months long.

Meanwhile, Finn was taking daily doses of children's paracetamol, a painkiller, as well as antibiotics to fight a tooth abscess.[139] His face became "swollen like a chipmunk," according to his mother, who feared further complications.[140] "I feel very bad a lot of the time and it hurts me especially when I want to go to sleep. I hope a dentist man can make it go away soon," said Finn.[141]

Karen was desperate to find treatment for her son, who had to be taken out of school in the search for a dental appointment. She repeatedly made calls to the Weston Clinic that literally went unanswered. A return visit to the White Dental Spa surgery center yielded only faxed requests for an appointment in Manchester within 13 weeks time.[142] Paying up to 1,200 British pounds (~$1,950) out-of-pocket for private treatment was not a viable alternative for the single mother.[143] Karen was running out of options.

"What type of system is it that no one seems to care that a child is suffering for six months?" asks Karen. "This is an emergency but I cannot get anyone to accept responsibility, there is no accountability whatsoever. There seems to be no prioritization."[144]

Fortunately, local media exposure about Finn's months of suffering prompted faster action by the local health authorities, Cheshire Primary Care Trust. In April 2006, at last, dentists removed Finn's two aching teeth.[145]

Though relieved that her son is no longer in pain, Karen remarked, "[I]t is a shame that I had to go to such extremes to get treatment for Finn, after all he just needed a tooth out. I feel sorry for the other boys and girls suffering the same way. The waiting list for people in pain should never have got to that level."[146]

MOTHER DELIVERS BABY IN HOSPITAL BATHROOM WITH ONLY HER OWN MOTHER TO HELP

Catherine Brown, 30, of Hornchurch, England was forced to deliver her 18-weeks-old (22 weeks premature) baby in a hospital bathroom with only her mother by her side because there was not qualified staff on hand to assist.[147]

On the evening of February 21, 2007, Brown was rushed to Queen's Hospital in Essex after she began hemorrhaging. She was stabilized with intravenous antibiotics and given a bed in the hospital's general mixed-sex ear, nose and throat division, instead of in a maternity ward. The newly-built, nearly half a billion dollar state-of-the-art hospital did not have a dedicated gynecology division.[148]

Brown was promised a scan the next morning to determine the health of her baby. However, by 5 pm the next day, she had not received it. After Brown's infuriated mother, Sheila Keeling, threatened to complain officially, doctors administered a scan that evening – over 20 hours since Brown's arrival at the hospital. The scan revealed there was no amniotic fluid surrounding the baby.[149] Doctors advised, and Brown agreed, to induce labor because the baby had a slight chance of survival and Brown's life was at risk, according to doctors.[150]

"I had no idea whether my baby was dead or alive. I was very ill. They gave me a pill to induce labor. I was put in a side room with my mum on my own and went into labor," recalled Brown.[151]

Roughly four hours after taking the pill, Brown went into labor at 4 am. Yet, with no trained medical staff to meaningfully assist, Brown was left to stand over a toilet in the hospital bathroom. At 8 am on February 23, Brown gave birth to Edward Paul in a bedpan the staff provided.[152] The premature baby died minutes after the horrific delivery.[153]

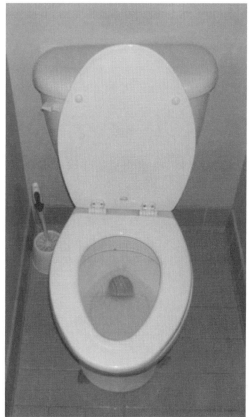

Credit: Ryan Balis

Thanks to a staff shortage, Catherine Brown was forced to deliver her premature baby in a hospital bathroom with only her mother assisting.

"When I delivered him, I just howled and howled," said Brown. "It was pure distress. He was still attached to the umbilical cord and I remember just looking at him and thinking 'What do I do next?' Then I started crying and just saying 'Sorry, baby, I'm so sorry.'"[154]

Sheila Keeling, the mother, recalled her daughter's terrifying delivery:

> Catherine was left to deliver the baby alone with just me for help before cleaning herself up and going back to bed. It was horrific. I was running around frantically for over an hour trying to find gas and air for her, and pleaded with nurses, who seemed very matter of fact, to come and assist. The staff I did find told me they didn't have the training to help.[155]

Brown added, "There were no staff that could help. They were all very good but they were not the gynecological ward so they didn't know what to do. They did their best but it was like a plumber tying to do an electrician's job."[156]

But Brown's nightmare was not over. In addition to the details of Edward's birth not being recorded by the hospital, to her horror, the baby's body was nearly disposed of with medical waste. The family instructed hospital staff that they wished to have the body released for a burial, but an administrative mistake almost led to it being wrongfully discarded.[157]

According to a spokesman for the government-managed National Health Service at the Barking, Havering and Redbridge Trust, since Brown's ordeal it has made improvements:

> We have now established a separate gynecological A&E [Accident and Emergency] service, staffed by gynecological, medical and nursing staff with access to the Early Pregnancy Assessment Unit. From the end of this month, there will be a dedicated gynecological ward, with the Early Pregnancy Assessment Unit situated within it. This will ensure dedicated and appropriate care.[158]

Despite steps to ensure that a situation similar to Brown's experience is not repeated, Brown is amazed at the lack of care she received. "I still can't believe the hospital had no trained staff who could help me," she said.[159]

MOM OF CHOKING BABY TOLD TO WAIT 35 MINUTES FOR AMBULANCE

It was any parent's worst fear. Nicola Cook's eight-week-old daughter, Scarlett, was choking to death.

"I was tapping her on the back and could not hear any breathing coming out,"[160] said Cook, 29, from Okehampton, England.[161] "I was trying to help her but her eyes started to go red and she was struggling to breathe."[162]

Frantically, Cook, who lives one mile from a hospital, dialed emergency services only to be told an ambulance would arrive in 35 minutes.

"When I called 999 [the emergency telephone number], the man said the ambulance was on its way and it was only when I pressed him he said it would take 35 minutes," said Cook.[163]

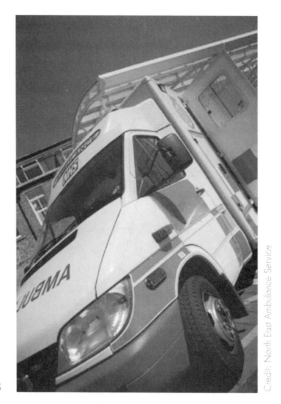

When eight-week-old Scarlett Cook wasn't breathing, Britain's NHS said it would send an ambulance in 35 minutes.

Cook recalls that the emergency operator asked if Scarlett was on her side, but was otherwise not helpful. "The general impression I got was that he was quite keen to get off the phone... I was panicking and telling him she was not breathing and was going to die. I was smacking her on the back and she started taking in air in fits and starts."[164]

Frantically, Cook asked a neighbor, Kath Taylor, for a car ride to the Okehampton Community Hospital, one mile away. At the hospital, Scarlett was treated with emergency oxygen.[165] "Fortunately the hospital was open until 10 pm but what if this had happened at night?" asked Cook.[166]

Doctors at Okehampton then sent Scarlett to the Royal Devon and Exeter Hospital for further evaluation of her breathing difficulties and treatment. Thankfully, Scarlett recovered fully.[167]

Cook explained what had affected Scarlett's breathing:

> They told me that Scarlett had been choking on milk and that it had gone
> back into her lungs. She was getting air by this time but her breathing was
> still up and down. They put a monitor on her finger and said her oxygen
> levels were low. The doctors were brilliant and told me I had done the right
> thing in bringing her as soon as possible. I don't know what would have
> happened if I'd waited. I was convinced she was dying.[168]

Cook should have received speedier emergency service, according to Britain's own
government health targets. They set a target of exactly eight minutes or less for an
ambulance to reach "immediately life threatening" calls.[169] Moreover, Kevin Lyons,
branch secretary of the Ambulance Service Union, acknowledged, "In this case, an
eight-week-old baby choking should have been classed as a life-threatening incident
and a vehicle should have been there within eight minutes."[170]

But Cook's sparse town of Okehampton has only one ambulance to serve it, which
Lyons confirms.

"At Okehampton they have one ambulance and when that is out they are sent
one from Crediton or Exeter [about a half hour away]," he says. "Other towns
like Ivybridge and Teignmouth don't even have an ambulance. With the system
as it is, there is always the possibility that someone will die as a result of
waiting too long."[171]

THANKS TO NURSE SHORTAGE, BABY BORN IN PARKING LOT

Sally West was forced to deliver her daughter, Phoebe, in the back of an ambulance
because of a public hospital's nurse shortage.

West was due to give birth at Malton Community Hospital, which is three miles
from her home in North Yorkshire, England. When West began to go into labor,
an ambulance and an on-call nurse were called to her home. But instead of being
taken on a short trip to nearby Malton, West was told she could not be booked there
because the local hospital did not have any nurses on hand. Instead, the on-call
nurse examined West and determined there was enough time before delivery to send
her to the larger Scarborough Hospital, 25 miles away.[172]

But half an hour into being transferred to the alternate hospital, West went into labor while still in the ambulance and without a nurse present.[173] With no time to move West inside the hospital, ambulance paramedics riding along with West were left to deliver the baby in the hospital's parking lot.[174]

Irritated, West said, "I really wanted to have my baby in Malton because it's so homely there and, after all, it's my home-town hospital."[175] "It [was] appalling. We are lucky everything turned out OK. It could have been a very different story."[176]

Explaining the astounding circumstances, she added:

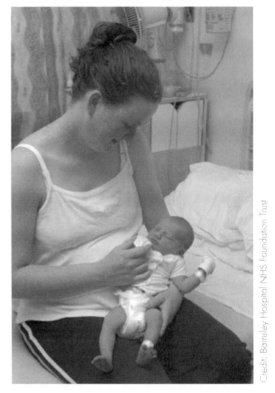

Thanks to a nurse shortage, Sally West delivered baby Phoebe in an ambulance (models shown).

> The midwife could not hang around with me because she was on call. I do not blame the midwife because, had she known I was about to give birth I am sure she would have stayed with me, but thinking I was okay and had plenty of time she packed me off to Scarborough… But the baby came along much quicker than expected and I ended up having the baby in the car park of the hospital just half-an-hour later.[177]

Thankfully, Phoebe was born healthy and without further complication, but Clive Milson, West's partner, unfortunately missed the birth of his daughter. He was following behind the ambulance during the ordeal. He described the scene as "just a debacle – a nightmare situation."[178] Milson continued, "It's easy to lose a life in a situation like this. I thank my lucky stars that our little girl was delivered safe and well, even if it was in a car park in the back of an ambulance."[179]

A spokesperson from the regional health authority, Scarborough and North East Yorkshire Healthcare NHS Trust, offered an explanation: "[U]nfortunately it isn't safe to deliver babies if we're having difficulty with staffing levels, which can be quite difficult to maintain in a small unit. Some babies do arrive more quickly than expected, and it can be better to deliver in an ambulance than attempt to move mum at a late stage," said Gilly Collinson, the trust's communication manger.[180]

ALL THE SOCIALIZED MEDICINE YOU WON'T GET

James Tyndale of Cambridge, England fought the National Health Service to get a life-extending cancer drug that was available under the NHS to cancer patients elsewhere in Britain but not in his locality.

For Tyndale, who is referred to here by a pseudonym, surviving terminal bone marrow cancer appeared unlikely. Treatment, which had included a stem cell transplant and Thalidomide, failed to weaken the cancer, and doctors gave him only months to live. Tyndale's last hope, doctors said, was Velcade, an expensive yet powerful drug.[181] The treatment would cost about £15,000 (~$24,400) and could extend Tyndale's life up to two years if successful.[182]

The problem was Tyndale's local health provider, Cambridge City Primary Care Trust, which refused to pay for Velcade because of its high cost, although it is available in other British cities under the government's health service.[183] This geographical health care variance is referred to as the NHS "postcode lottery," in which there are significant differences in access to care and treatment depending on one's postcode, or locality.[184]

"There's clear evidence of significant geographical variation," said Joanne Rule, chief executive of CancerBacup, an information and support charity for cancer victims. "The trusts won't pay for anything until it has been fully authorized by NICE [the government's health adviser], but even when that happens, there is no one whose responsibility it is to say that prescribing those drugs must happen. This is beginning to impact on people's chances of survival."[185]

It outraged Tyndale, as well as doctors,[186] that the NHS was denying Tyndale a drug that could slow his cancer and prolong his life.

"It is appalling that patients whose thoughts should be focused on their treatment need to waste time worrying about how to obtain the drugs which will give them a last lifeline. For these vital drugs, we need countrywide consistency," argued Tyndale.[187]

Facing imminent death, Tyndale enlisted the assistance of his parliamentarian and the Tory Shadow Health Secretary, MP Andrew Lansley.[188] "I have put it to the PCT [the NHS health provider] that they should make Velcade available... but they are still to come back to me," said Lansley.[189]

That even a national politician would be stonewalled, Tyndale observed, "I feel that I'm caught in a game of bureaucratic tennis. I don't know the rules of the game, but I know my life is at stake."[190]

But Tyndale's persistence paid off. At last, the health provider authorized funding for Tyndale's treatment, and in May 2006, Tyndale received Velcade.[191]

DOCTORS REFUSE FOOT SURGERY ON MAN BECAUSE HE SMOKES

John Nuttall of Cornwall, England is in a showdown with the government-managed British National Health Service. An NHS hospital refused to treat his shattered ankle unless he stopped smoking cigarettes.[192]

Nuttall, 57, fractured his ankle in three places after falling off a ladder while on the job in 2005.[193] Because Nuttall worried that surgery would result in further complications, a plaster cast was used to immobilize the fractured bones. After six months, though, the ankle had not healed naturally, and, Nuttall said, he was left to "beg" doctors to revisit the surgery option.[194]

But, said Nuttall, the doctors' "attitude was completely changed."[195] Doctors at Royal Cornwall Hospital told Nuttall they would not operate unless he quit his 20-cigarette a day habit. They said a smoker's bones would not stand as good a chance of healing and there was a risk of needing amputation after surgery if complications developed.[196] They provided Nuttall with a Northwestern University Medical School study that found 68 percent of the 54 smoking patients it studied fully recovered from a similar surgery done on the wrist, compared to 95 percent of non-smokers.[197]

A spokesperson at Royal Cornwall explained that the delay hinged on nicotine levels: "Smoking has a big influence on this surgery. The healing process will be significantly hindered."[198] The doctors' decision came mere months after then-Health Secretary Patricia Hewitt authorized a NHS policy that smokers can be

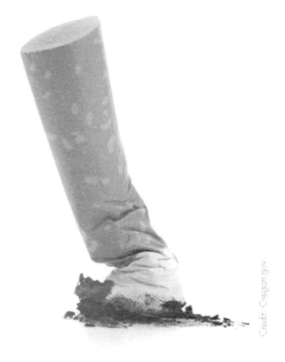

Britain's NHS won't operate on John Nuttall's shattered ankle because he smokes cigarettes.

denied non-life threatening operations, unless a blood test confirms they quit for at least four weeks in advance.[199]

For Nuttall, postponed surgery means continuing life in constant pain. "I'm in agony. I can feel the bones grating… I've begged them to operate but they won't. I've tried my hardest to give up smoking but I can't. I got down to ten a week but they said that wasn't good enough."[200]

Before they would rebuild the ankle, doctors wanted Nuttall to pledge not to smoke for three months following surgery.[201]

Meanwhile, for years, Nuttall took daily doses of prescription morphine to dull the pain, and used a cane to get around on his good foot.[202] Because of the morphine, he would not drive.[203]

"I have paid my dues as a taxpayer – and now the NHS won't treat me," said a frustrated Nuttall.[204] Worse yet, he feared surgery might not improve his ankle at this late stage. "The bones have all calcified now – it's probably too late for surgery but I want other smokers in my age group to know that we are being denied medical treatment and there's nothing we can do."[205]

NO BEDS AT HOSPITAL, SO BABY BORN AT HOME

A public hospital in Britain left Julia Evans of Brighton to deliver her baby at home, with no midwife present. The birth occurred just hours after the hospital refused to allow her to stay at the hospital.

The reason? No beds were available.[206]

In early August 2007, a pregnant Evans arrived at Royal Sussex County Hospital in deep pain. She was overdue for delivery and believed she was going into labor. Nevertheless, the hospital would not admit Evans because it did not have any beds available. A junior doctor who examined Evans insisted she was not going into labor and sent her home.

A National Health Service spokesperson later explained that Evans was not believed to be in "established labor" because the doctor did not observe any blood.

Evans, who is a former medical representative herself, recalled, "I was in so much agony and pain but you trust doctors to do and know what is right. They kept saying I was not in labor, but I was."

Hours later, now at home, Evans' water broke. A friend called the hospital, but doctors refused to send a midwife, insisting there was time before she delivered the baby. In desperation, they called an ambulance, and paramedics helped Evans deliver. But her troubles were about to get worse.

The paramedics on site were not permitted to cut the umbilical cord. The hospital was called but again said no midwife was available to come to Evans' aid. The ambulance would have to take her in to the hospital to be detached and monitored. Thus, with umbilical cord still attached, the 37-year-old mother was forced to carry her newborn down the stairs of her home to the waiting ambulance.

"I'm disgusted at how I was treated," said Evans. "They should have more midwives available and on call to come out when there is an emergency."

Thankfully, the baby was born healthy, but Evans developed complications and an infection and returned to the hospital for two days of intravenous antibiotics. Though recovered physically, the hellish home delivery left Evans so traumatized that only after four weeks of coping was she able to name her son, Harvey.

"I feel like I lost out on the first week of my son's life because I went through so much," said Evans. "If I did not have a friend with me at the time I dread to think what might have happened."

Evans is currently pursuing legal action over her nightmarish experience with the NHS. "I don't want people to have to go through the same thing as me," she said.

FOUR-HOUR WAIT FOR BURN VICTIM

Ernest Smith of Blackburn, England faced a four-hour wait in a hospital emergency room for treatment of severe burns he suffered because of a gas explosion.[207]

Smith, who by occupation is a driller, mistakenly punctured a camp stove oven on which he was working. Observing a small flame, Smith opened the oven, which allowed emitted gas to ignite into a fireball.

Smith's hair and eyebrows were torched and his arms badly burned. An ambulance

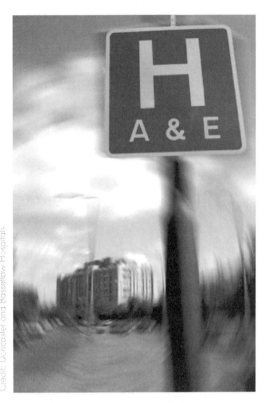

Credit: Doncaster and Bassetlaw Hospitals

After he received severe burns from a gas explosion, Ernest Smith faced a four-hour wait in a NHS Accident & Emergency Center.

rushed him to the accident and emergency (A&E) center at Royal Blackburn Hospital – a government-managed hospital within the British National Health Service. But upon his arrival at the emergency room, despite Smith's agony, hospital staff provided Smith only with medication. They told him he'd have to wait for treatment until doctors took care of 12 already waiting patients, a wait which was estimated to take up to four hours.

"I'd been there for an hour already and got up to see what was going on," Smith explained. "I spotted a lot of nurses sitting around a table not treating people, and was told that I might have to wait up to four hours before I could be seen."

Infuriated and not certain when doctors would get to his burns, Smith left the hospital to seek care on his own. However, it would not be several days before his swollen and blistered arms were treated at a local surgery center.

Though NHS guidelines specify patients in an emergency department should be treated within four hours,[208] Smith is disgusted with his experience. "[I] was in quite a lot of pain and think it's scandalous that I couldn't see anyone," he said.

Despite the poor quality of hospital service, an NHS employee seemed to place blame on Smith for not receiving adequate treatment. "The patient in question was seen within 15 minutes of arrival and given medication within 20 minutes. In under an hour the patient had decided to leave under his own accord without the completion of his treatment," said Lynda Walker, A&E service manager of the East Lancashire Hospitals NHS Trust.

NO HOSPITAL BEDS FOR MOTHER'S BABY

Early one morning, a pregnant Adele Wake of Milnsbridge, England was rushed to the hospital in labor.[209] Though her baby was 11 weeks premature, Wake was scheduled to give birth at Calderdale Royal Hospital in nearby Halifax. However, when Wake arrived there at 1:20 am Saturday, she learned the hospital did not have neo-natal beds available.

Moreover, not only was Calderdale short of beds, so too was the nearest alternative facility, Huddersfield Royal Infirmary. Instead, Wake, while in labor, would be transferred 30 miles away to a third hospital.

At 10 am, an ambulance transferred Wake to Jessops Hospital in Sheffield. Because of traffic conditions, the 30-mile trip took an hour and ten minutes. Fortunately, Wake held off immediate delivery, giving birth to a 3 pound, 2 ounce baby boy named Joseph that following Monday. Nevertheless, moving hospitals during delivery upset the family.

"It was an ordeal for my wife and very stressful for me. If Joseph had arrived while they were in the ambulance he might not be here now," said Wake's husband, Roy Wake. "The situation has disgusted us and our whole family. They can't believe we had to be transferred while Adele was in labor."

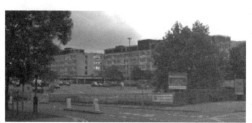

Because of Joseph's premature birth, he was put on support machines at the hospital. The Wakes were told they would not be able to take Joseph back to Milnsbridge for 10 weeks.

Roy Wake continued, "We want to get him home, but we have to wait for a space at Halifax. It makes it difficult really and it's a stressful time."

All full at Huddersfield Royal Infirmary when Adele Wake arrived in labor.

Following the ordeal, Helen Thomson, director of nursing for the Calderdale and Huddersfield NHS Trust, explained the bed shortage. "That day there was an unusually high demand for our intensive care cots and they were all occupied. A baby born 10 weeks early should always be delivered in a centre with an intensive care cot."

But a shortage of beds situation may continue. The Calderdale Royal and Huddersfield Royal have a combined total of only six intensive care neo-natal beds.

SIX PERCENT OF BRITONS RESORT TO DO-IT-YOURSELF DENTISTRY

Self-dentistry appears to be a way of life for many in Britain. British newspapers tell of Britons who are unable to locate a dentist on the government's National

Health Service removing their own teeth, scraping plaque off with screwdrivers, and even attaching their own crowns, using superglue.[210]

When the NHS failed to treat him, Don Wilson of Kent, England's method of choice for relieving a toothache was using fishing pliers to pull it. Wilson attempted to see a dentist to have his rotting teeth professionally removed, but was unsuccessful at locating a public dentist.[211]

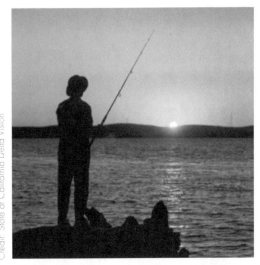

Don Wilson used a tool designed to get a hook out of a fish's mouth to remove five of his own teeth when Britain's public health service couldn't provide him with a dentist (model shown).

"When you've got a severe toothache, you don't want to wait two or three weeks – you need treatment straightaway... But when I used to ring up dentists, either they couldn't see me on the NHS for weeks, or had no NHS patients at all," he said.[212]

A visit to a local hospital's emergency room also proved unsuccessful. Because hospital staff would not extract his teeth, in desperation, Wilson decided he would perform the job himself. He explained:

I went for a rummage around in my tool box and found these fishing disgorgers – the tool you use to get a hook out of the back of a fish's mouth... I thought: "These will do the job," and just started pulling it out. Obviously there's no anesthetic, and it's very painful, but you just shut it out and get on with it."[213]

Wilson continued, describing in detail, "I sit at my desk to do it, and when my wife comes in, she just grimaces at what I'm doing... It takes a few minutes, and you keep pulling and pulling, then you get this cracking sound, and the tooth just comes out."[214]

Wilson has attempted to remove five of his teeth (one such tooth broke in half and remains stuck in his gum) using this homemade method. In fact, tooth extraction is not the only reason for which Wilson has turned to his toolkit.[215]

"If I've got a hole in my tooth, and it's hurting, I'll put a heated needle in the hole and that just kills the nerve, and stops the pain," Wilson explained. "I've also used liquid metal adhesive to stick crowns back on."[216]

Alarmingly, such makeshift dental work is not unique in the UK. A thorough 2007 survey of over 5,200 dental patients in Britain by the Commission for Patient and

Public Involvement in Health found six percent of those questioned – or more than one out of every 20 – had resorted to some form of dental self-treatment, which can involve pulling one's own teeth.[217] One such respondent from Lancashire extracted 14 of his own teeth by using pliers.[218] Another in Essex used "modified tweezers" to remove "jagged bits" of tooth after this patient's dentist could not schedule an emergency appointment.[219]

The British paper Daily Express commented that such a gruesome do-it-yourself practice is "a damning indictment of a [NHS] system harking back to the Victorian era..."[220] In fact, the British government estimates that more than two million people who wish to have publicly-done treatment cannot access a NHS dentist.[221] Moreover, some patients wait up to one year just to register with a NHS dentist.[222]

When it comes to home-done dentistry, Don Wilson apparently speaks for many Britons: "If you're in agony with toothache, you haven't got much choice."[223]

LONG DENTIST WAIT OR PULL SEVEN OF OWN TEETH?

The dilemma facing Arthur Haupt of Leicestershire, England was this choice: Should he wait three weeks for a government dentist to relieve a painful toothache or pay hundreds of pounds for private dental care out-of-pocket?

For Haupt, a 67-year-old cab driver and Army veteran,[224] neither choice was acceptable. Instead, he performed the job himself by pulling out his own teeth.

In December 2006, Haupt visited ADP NHS Dental Practice in Melton. Despite Haupt's agony, staff told Haupt to fill out paperwork and to come back in three weeks.[225]

"When they told me to fill out a form and how long I would have to wait I said 'I've got gob ache now, not in three weeks time," said Haupt. "It's rubbish isn't it. When you say you've got bad toothache you expect them to say 'Yeah, we'll see you today or tomorrow.'"[226]

A private dentist Haupt consulted off the National Health Service quoted him a price of £75 (~$122) per tooth pulled,[227] which would total nearly £55 (~$1,200) for the seven teeth Haupt needed removed. Haupt considered the sum unaffordable.

"If you can't get anyone else to take your teeth out you take them out yourself don't

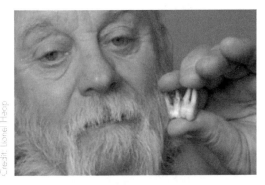

Arthur Haupt's toothache was so painful, he said it felt "like a knife going through my eye." When the NHS said a dental appointment would take three weeks, he pulled his teeth out himself.

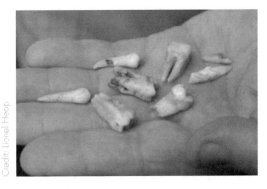

Arthur Haupt extracted these seven teeth at home with pliers. Six percent of Britons have resorted to some form of self-dentistry.

you," he said, matter-of-factly. "I had raging toothache. It was like a knife going through my eye."[228]

Haupt explained the do-it-yourself technique he learned while in the Army in gruesome detail. "I went home, got some pliers, got hold of the tooth and twisted... I pulled it and out it came, and all this black, smelly yuck came out. [But w]ithin an hour my headache had gone."[229]

Over the next several weeks, Haupt yanked out an additional six loose teeth himself.[230] "There's a bit of pain at first, but it was nothing like the pain I was in when I first went to the dentist...," he said.[231] His wife, Sylvia, said, "I couldn't bear to watch him do it. It took some guts."[232]

Haupt joked that he had so many extracted teeth that he could line them up on display or make a necklace out of them.[233]

Commenting on Haupt's self-dental treatment, Howard Watkinson, chairman of the Leicestershire local dental committee, said, "It's a sad reflection on NHS provision that someone feels the need to resort to treating themselves which, at the very least is unsatisfactory and, at worst, could be dangerous."[234]

But Haupt is not alone. Valerie Holsworth, a 67-year-old great-grandmother from Scarborough, also used pliers along with beer and whiskey as anesthesia to pull seven of her own bothersome teeth.[235] "I'm not a masochist but the job needed doing," Holsworth said. "It is just a matter of tugging and wiggling until the root comes loose."[236]

A national survey of over 5,200 dental patients in the UK discovered that, alarmingly, some six percent resort to some type of do-it-yourself dental work.[237] Without an available dentist, many are resorting, primitively, to pulling their own teeth.[238]

REFUSED EMERGENCY CARE, WOMAN RIPS OUT AGONIZING TOOTH WITH FINGERNAILS

Susannah Houghton of Radcliffe, England awoke one Saturday morning with an agonizing toothache. She was in so much pain she could not eat, sleep or even open her mouth to talk properly.[239] But the government-run National Health Service refused her emergency dental treatment because she had not been in pain long enough.

"The pain was so bad it was driving me mad," Houghton said. "I wanted to bang my head against the wall – anything to distract me from the pain – I've had four children and I've never experienced anything like this."[240]

That Saturday, Houghton contacted her local after-hours dental NHS service, Bury and Rochdale Doctors On Call. Houghton said she pleaded – in fact, "begged" – for urgent relief.[241] But NHS staff decided the situation did not warrant emergency service because "I had not been in pain for at least 48 hours," Houghton explained.[242] Instead, she was told to call back on Monday.[243]

Tormented by pain and rejected by the NHS, Houghton became desperate. "I begged them to help me, but when they wouldn't I had to do something to help myself," she said. "I knew there was a chance I could cause an infection or have complications but the pain put those fears to the back of my mind."[244]

By Saturday evening, Houghton could no longer tolerate the pain and decided to pull out the broken tooth using her artificial fingernails.[245] "I wriggled the tooth around until I felt it crack," she described. "My mum told me not to do it in case I bled to death but I just could not cope any longer. I felt like jumping off a cliff."[246]

On Sunday, Houghton went to the emergency room and was given antibiotics. She would have to wait until Tuesday to have the root of the aching tooth removed.[247]

"I know I'm not the only person to be driven to this, [but] there is something very wrong with a system which leaves you in pain and without help," she said.[248]

Anthony Halperrin of the Patients' Association, a UK health care charity, was equally disturbed about Britons having to resort to self-dentistry. "It's simply astonishing that in this day and age we have people pulling their own teeth out."[249]

Yet, trouble finding a dentist is not uncommon in Britain's rationed-care system.

For instance, in parts of the southwest, patients must travel long distances of 40, 50 or 75 miles for dental treatment – that is, if they are lucky enough to find a dentist still accepting patients under the NHS.[250] In Scunthorpe, some patients wait more than four years for specialist treatment.[251] Nationwide, other patients needing extensive work, such as multiple fillings, crowns and repeat visits, are turned away by public dentists who say they cannot afford to treat patients who need extensive work thanks to the way government payment policies are structured.[252]

"IN BRITAIN... I FELT LIKE A LUMP OF MEAT ON THE PRODUCTION LINE"

Russ Aiton, a long-time supporter of the British National Health Service, never expected to fly 5,000 miles from his native England when he needed surgery to save his life.[253]

Aiton, a former medical consultant for a NHS children's hospital in Sheffield, found his confidence in the government's health service shaken when he was warned he would need to wait several months for an urgently-needed heart bypass operation.

"I was diagnosed 18 months ago with heart disease and chronic atrial fibrillation – an irregular heartbeat – and my condition soon began to [get] worse," Aiton, then 43, said. "I couldn't walk up stairs, I couldn't travel for my work, I couldn't lift anything and I was putting on weight. Effectively I was in heart failure."

Afraid to take the chance the NHS wouldn't offer care while his heart was still beating, Aiton and his wife, Joy, searched for another option.

"[W]hen I found out I would have to wait several months for an operation, despite my consultant at Aberdeen hospital saying I needed an urgent heart bypass, Joy and I decided we had to go private," he explained.

After a brief Internet search, Aiton discovered the Taj Medical Group. The independent company offered to get Aiton the surgery and recuperation he needed in Bangalore, India within weeks. The surgery would cost the couple thousands of pounds out-of-pocket and require extensive travel, but Aiton faced possible death if he waited for the NHS to get around to providing the care he was entitled to as a contributor.

Thus, in September 2007, Aiton and his wife flew to India. The operation was carried out successfully at Wockhardt Hospital in Bangalore, and soon thereafter Aiton was well enough to return to work. "I've been given a new lease of life and I feel bloody marvelous," Aiton exclaimed.

Aiton praised the quality of care he received in India. "Nothing was too much trouble for the staff. The care, the cleanliness and the attention to detail were all excellent," he said. "There was no comparison to my treatment in Britain, where I felt like a lump of meat on the production line." Aiton added, "I'm sorry to say Third World standards are what we now find in British hospitals."

Apparently, tens of thousands of Britons who are stuck on waiting lists or afraid of contracting disease in a public hospital agree. As some foreign health centers offer timely care at a fraction of domestic private rates in Britain, an estimated 100,000 Britons traveled abroad for medical, dental and cosmetic treatments in 2007 alone.[254] The number of these so-called "health tourists" in the UK is expected to increase to 200,000 by the end of 2010.[255]

To meet growing demand, Britain's first health tourism exhibition was held in London in October 2008 to promote medical treatments and health facilities abroad.[256]

"AN ANIMAL WOULD HAVE BEEN TREATED WITH MORE COMPASSION"

Ian Luck spent the last weeks of his life in agony because of a complete lack of care at the government-run Princess Alexandra Hospital in Essex, UK, where he died in 2002."[257]

For over five years, Luck's widow, Debra, and nine-year-old son, Ben, fought for answers as to why hospital staff neglected Luck, frequently leaving him to lay in his own vomit and waste and failing to realize the severity of his increasingly-desperate state.

Luck checked in to the Princess Alexandra on June 12, 2002 after being too weak to eat and vomiting heavily. He had suffered for several years from gastric problems and was treated twice in 2002 for lost fluids because of vomiting and diarrhea. This time, an endoscope discovered an ulcer. Doctors prescribed antibiotics to Luck, gave him fluids and sent him home after a six-day stay.

On June 20, Luck returned to the hospital for a second endoscope exam when the inflammation in his stomach had not cleared up. However, the ulcer ruptured during the procedure, and emergency surgery had to be performed to repair it.

Following surgery, Debra Luck was effectively left to look after his health and comfort.

"No one wanted to help us. Every time we asked for pain relief, or to see a doctor, we were told to wait, or that we didn't know what we were talking about," she said.

Luck's condition continued to decline, but hospital staff showed an utter lack of sympathy. Debra Luck recalled that the staff failed to or were slow to perform basic functions, such as cleaning up after her husband.

"He was vomiting ten times an hour, and there were bowls around his bed to catch it," she said. However, "Often they weren't emptied for more than an hour and they smelled awful. The first time that happened I found a nurse and asked if she could empty them. When she said she was too busy, I offered to do it myself."

Debra Luck began resorting to bringing in clean pillowcases, shirts and pants, and having to change her husband herself. "As fast as I changed him he was sick again. The nurses were not interested in helping me," she said. "An animal would have been treated with more compassion."

Meanwhile, it was not known if the bleeding from the ulcer had stopped. "I made two appointments to speak to a consultant during the course of those ten days," she said, "and both times he didn't turn up. When I tried to talk to junior doctors, they were either too busy or didn't know enough."

Frustrated and fearing for her husband's life, Debra Luck attempted to have Ian transferred to a local private hospital. Though the private hospital agreed, staff at the Princess Alexandra rejected the move because Luck was not stable.

On June 28, at the request of a junior doctor, a consultant at last saw Luck. But the consultant failed to follow up on the suggestion that a laparotomy (surgical examination), which might have determined the definitive cause of Luck's bleeding, be carried out. On June 29, a second junior doctor called for a consultant's review, which was never performed.

Two days later, after a particularly agonizing night in which nurses forgot to inject painkillers, Luck began to lapse in and out of consciousness and struggle to breathe. That morning, "He was covered in vomit and had wet himself," remembered Debra. "I changed him, but when I asked for clean surgical stockings the nurse said there were none left in his size... I couldn't change his T-shirt without help... but I was told by the nurse she was too busy and to leave him dirty."

That evening, a junior doctor suspected that Luck had suffered a collapsed lung and ordered a chest X-ray. But Luck went into cardiac arrest during the procedure and had to be resuscitated. By the time family members arrived, Luck already suffered a second, fatal cardiac arrest.

"I actually feel that Ian was murdered," Debra said. "He died because people couldn't be bothered to do their job properly."

Debra Luck contends that the hospital did not carry out necessary tests. "What I've learned since is that his urine and vomit should have been monitored continuously. Both were vital to working out just how ill he was and whether he would need further investigations. The fact that no one kept a record probably added to his lack of correct treatment."

In October 2007, the Princess Alexandra Hospital NHS Trust agreed to compensate Debra and Ben a combined sum of £225,000 (~$366,000), though the National Health Service refused to accept liability for Luck's death.

For her part, Debra Luck remains angry, telling Britain's Daily Mail, "No one has been punished or sacked. No one from the hospital has offered to meet me and tell me how things went so wrong, let alone offered an apology. For all I know, the same appalling standard of care is still acceptable in that hospital. If that is the case, then there will be more unnecessary deaths."

ELDERLY MAN SPENDS LIFE SAVINGS FOR PRIVATE HIP REPLACEMENT AFTER NHS CANCELS FOUR APPOINTMENTS

Edward Crane, 75, of Essex, England emptied his bank account to pay for essential surgery because the government-run British National Health Service cancelled his appointment four times over a more than six-month period.[258]

In February 2007, doctors at Crane's local hospital outside London in Essex told him he needed hip replacement surgery. An X-ray performed in the emergency center revealed Crane was without a hip joint, according to Polly Taylor, Crane's daughter.

Doctors referred Crane to Queen's Hospital in Romford, but Queen's cancelled four consecutive appointments. In agony, Crane decided he had "no choice" but to use his own savings to pay for private surgery.

"It has been heartbreaking. He was in so much pain," said Taylor.

To pay for the expensive operation, Crane used two private insurance policies and withdrew all his savings. Four days after the last cancelled NHS appointment, a private surgeon carried out the operation. Though the surgery cost £8,750 (~$14,200), Taylor believes her father might have died if he had waited for the NHS to perform the surgery.

"If he hadn't had it done privately he would have died of the pain," she said. "He has nothing left now. It's not fair how the NHS treats old people."

Because Crane had the surgery done privately, it is unlikely that the NHS will reimburse his expenses – despite the emergency situation. "It is extremely unlikely that anyone would be able to claim back money from the NHS if they chose to be treated privately," said a spokesman for Barking, Havering and Redbridge NHS Trust.

Under Britain's rationed care health system, the length of Crane's wait is not unusual. The average wait time for a hip replacement is six months in the Barking, Havering and Redbridge NHS Trust jurisdiction.

Nationwide, according to the NHS's own figures, some 37,600 patients waited 12 months or more just to go to a NHS hospital in 2007.[259]

12-MINUTE AMBULANCE RIDE TAKES NEARLY THREE HOURS - EVERY TIME

Morris Howard requires four hours of dialysis three times per week.[260] Since April 2007, when his kidneys failed and were removed, Howard, 85, is taken by ambulance to the Royal Free Hospital to receive the life-saving treatment. The roughly mile-and-a-half journey to his home in Finchley, England should take 12 minutes by car.

Instead of a quick ride, under the National Health Service the elderly man is stuck inside an ambulance with other patients waiting to be dropped off for up to three hours per trip. After the demanding treatment at the hospital leaves Howard feeling sick and disoriented, the delay on the way home is especially taxing.

"Having to wait all that time to get home when I live so near made me very angry and the anger made me even more ill – it's very dangerous," explained Howard. "At the end of the dialysis… the last thing you want is to spend hours in an ambulance."

Moreover, the ambulance provided by National Ambulance Service, a private patient transporter under NHS contract, does not clearly specify when an ambulance will arrive to bring Howard to the hospital. Consequently, Howard must wake up at 5:30 am so as not to miss the ambulance.

"The people who run the ambulance service couldn't care a tinker's cuss about people who are sick and elderly," an outraged Howard exclaimed.

Fed up and exhausted from what he called an unreliable and haphazard ambulance service, Howard began to pay out-of-pocket for a taxi to take him home. For one year of treatment, he estimated the taxi cost at £1,000 pounds (~$1,600).

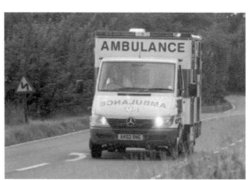

"The [ambulance] transport is very unreliable and haphazard," Howard said. "We are often told we have to wait for an ambulance to be available, and it's an absolute killer. How can they do this to human beings?"

The NHS used an ambulance to transport Morris Howard, 85, to and from his thrice-weekly dialysis treatments. The mile-and-a-half ride took nearly three hours each time.

Howard is not the only kidney patient experiencing a long wait. A 2007 report by the Nottingham University Hospitals Patient and Public Involvement Forum found that others being transported by the East Midlands Ambulance Service for dialysis waited up to four hours to be transported home from Nottingham City Hospital. In some cases, the report claimed, the hospital sent out a vehicle to pick up patients who had died.[261]

HOSPITAL TREATS ELDERLY MAN LIKE AN ANIMAL

Jenny Pitman of Berkshire, England is furious over the treatment her late father, George Harvey, received at a government-managed hospital.

Pitman said she was shocked over the "uncaring and mismanaged" hospital's lack of cleanliness and hygiene,[262] where, she maintains, Harvey contracted a bug that soon killed him.[263]

In November 2006, Harvey, 92, checked in to the Great Western Hospital in Wiltshire complaining of stomach pain. What ailed him, doctors believed, was a stomach ulcer, which blocked part of the intestine and prevented proper eating. Surgeons carried out a successful operation to bypass the blockage, and Harvey was given antibiotics. But when his condition began to deteriorate within a week of the operation, Pitman suspected something else was bothering her father that doctors had failed to treat.[264]

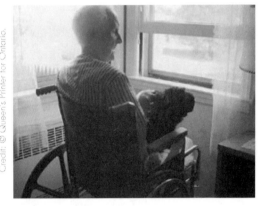

While admitted at a filthy NHS hospital, George Harvey contracted a deadly bacterium that his family maintains killed him (model shown).

"The blockage had been diagnosed as stomach cancer but the cancer was the size of a pea and hadn't spread," explained Pitman. "The reason he had become ill again was because he had contracted 'an infection' but we were never told what kind it was… [N]o one seemed unduly concerned."[265]

The mystery infection, unknown to the family at that time, was the deadly Clostridium Difficile (C. diff) bacterium known as the "superbug."[266] The infectious bug had invaded many of the UK's hospitals,[267] and has been linked to thousands of patient deaths.[268] As the bug progressed, Harvey became sicker. He was vomiting intensely, experiencing diarrhea and losing significant weight.[269]

"We could see he wasn't getting any better," Pitman recalled. "Yet, despite constantly asking staff why he wasn't recovering, no none seemed to notice or do anything about that fact that George was so unwell."[270]

Family members were left to sit by while Harvey's condition deteriorated further and to watch as hospital staff disgracefully neglected his care. "Once, my sister went in to find George lying half naked on a bedpan, on top of a bare mattress, with the sheets on the floor," said Pitman. "He was in agony and had been left like that for at least half an hour. Although he had desperately called for help, not one person had come to his aid."

"Another time," Pitman continued, "my husband David and I arrived at lunchtime to find him sat in bed, his cold, untouched shepherd's pie left on a trolley at the other end. George couldn't even reach it, yet no one had thought to check. Much of the time he was left not properly washed and stinking in a dirty bed. It is a dreadful illness and it had stripped George of all his dignity. He was humiliated and ashamed of himself, and although we told him it wasn't his fault he'd contracted this terrible illness, heartbreakingly, he thought it was."[271]

Despite the warning signs of a serious infection, hospital staff insisted on three occasions that Harvey had cancer and did not test even a stool sample for C. diff. Instead, after six weeks at the Great Western, Harvey was transferred to a hospice to receive round-the-clock care.[272]

"I cried the day he left that hospital," said Pitman. "But it wasn't only because I knew my father was making his final journey as he went into the hospice, it was also because I felt so relieved he was finally leaving such an uncaring and mismanaged place."[273]

At the Prospect Hospice,[274] staff suspected Harvey was infected with the superbug and isolated him in a private room.[275] He was diagnosed with the bug infection,[276] but tragically, Harvey was severely ill by this point and passed away two weeks later in early January 2007.[277]

Outraged, Pitman is currently compiling a list of "inexcusable shortfalls" at the Great Western and other National Health Service hospitals in a campaign demanding that they be cleaned up.[278] "We treat animals better than the NHS treat people in this country," she exclaimed.[279]

A statement released by the Great Western maintained Harvey died "from pneumonia and cancer" and there is "no evidence that he had Clostridium Difficile during his time at Great Western Hospital, nor was it associated with the cause of his death."[280] But a 2007 report by the Healthcare Commission, the former independent NHS watchdog,[281] revealed that between 90 and 270 patients died from C. diff at hospitals run by the Maidstone and Tunbridge Wells NHS Trust, which includes the Great Western. The report concluded: "[I]t is likely that *C. difficile* was definitely or probably the main cause of death in approximately 90 patients, and probably or definitely contributed to the deaths of approximately 270 patients between April 2004 and September 2006."[282]

HOSPITAL ADMITS NEW PATIENTS WHILE CURRENT ONES SUFFER

A government-managed hospital in Britain told Marilyn Townsend she would forgo her regularly-scheduled osteoporosis treatment for at least one year, allegedly so that other patients could be admitted in her place.[283]

Starting in 2003, the 75-year-old from Exning, England received pain relief injections, called a "diagnostic block," in her back every six months to a year at West Suffolk Hospital.[284] Townsend suffers from osteoporosis of the spine and found the injections effective at targeting the agonizing bone disorder.[285]

"I am just in pain all the time," she said. "It's getting worse and while the diagnostic blocks do not completely cure it, it puts the pain at bay."[286]

But in July 2007, Townsend was taken aback when, three days before her next treatment, she received a phone call that the appointment would be delayed for over one year – until at least August 2008 and perhaps as late as October 2008.[287]

"I thought they meant this August [2007]. But I was shocked when they said: 'No, it's next year,'" she explained.[288] "By then I will have been waiting two years."[289]

Townsend, a widow and retiree,[290] cannot afford private treatment and is forced to get by on tablets and patches, which burn her skin. Hoping to get her treatment resumed, she turned to her Member of Parliament, MP Richard Spring, who pressured Dr. Simon How, the general manager for medical services at West Suffolk, and the Department of Health.[291]

According to Spring, Townsend was overlooked because the hospital sought to meet National Health Service targets.[292] NHS guidelines state that new hospital patients should begin treatment within 18 weeks of a referral by a general practitioner.[293]

"It really is a profound bureaucratic misjudgment that the time period for new patients in practice pushes existing patients, who are suffering and in pain, into even greater discomfort," said Spring.[294] "This is a terrible case – the worst I have seen. It's bureaucracy gone mad."[295]

Smith's charge is supported by a doctor's letter rejecting a request to move up Townsend's treatment date. The Newmarket Journal reported:

> Although the hospital received a request from Mrs. Townsend's GP in Newmarket to move the appointment closer, a letter was sent back from consultant Dr. Rajesh Munglani, claiming it was unlikely it could be changed due to government pressure to focus on new patients and initial treatments.[296]

DO-IT-YOURSELF CHILDBIRTH – IN THE HOSPITAL

The last thing Annette Armstrong expected was that her own mother would be forced to deliver Armstrong's baby – inside a British maternity ward.[297] But Armstrong, her husband Daniel and Armstrong's mother were abandoned by the ward's preoccupied midwives, and had to handle the birth themselves.

Upon being admitted at a large maternity ward in Birmingham, Armstrong was alarmed that only two midwives were on duty to assist 10 women who either were in labor or who recently had delivered. One patient was a devastated mother who had given birth to a stillborn baby.

Armstrong described the chaos inside the ward. "The midwives were rushed off their feet and clearly couldn't meet the needs of all their patients. I got the feeling I was just a number, an item on a conveyor belt," she said.

Though she was in pain, Armstrong recalled that a midwife checked on her only once over a period of three hours. Husband Daniel tracked down an anesthetist to inject an epidural. The epidural should have numbed Armstrong's lower body, but the anesthetist botched it by injecting in the incorrect spot.

At last a different midwife appeared, but Armstrong was given what can only be described as a shoddy examination. "After a quick check she told me I wasn't progressing that quickly and it could be a while yet," she said. "Before I could ask any questions she was gone."

When the midwife returned, a second examination was equally incomplete. Again, the midwife insisted Armstrong was not in delivery, but, according to Armstrong, the midwife did not check how dilated she was. Instead, Armstrong said the midwife told her a trainee would come get her "if you really need me."

Soon thereafter, Armstrong was screaming that she was going into labor. "Daniel shouted at the trainee to get help, but she just stood in the corner looking petrified," Armstrong recalled. Armstrong's mom administered the delivery herself.

"My mum is not a midwife and I couldn't believe she was about to deliver my baby," exclaimed Armstrong. "Twenty minutes after the midwife had left, the baby was crowning – the top of its head had appeared. My mum said: 'This is your little girl and we have to get her out safely. There is no one else here to do this, so you have to trust me. Now start pushing.'"

Fortunately, Armstrong's mother managed to help her daughter deliver a healthy 8 lb. 9 oz. baby girl, Harriet.

"I couldn't believe the NHS staff had put us in that position," exclaimed Armstrong. "Were it not for my mum's advice and calm attitude, my child could have been starved of oxygen or had a whole host of other complications from not being delivered in time – she might even have died."

Armstrong's ordeal is not unique. According to a survey conducted by the Healthcare Commission, the former independent NHS watchdog,[298] 26 percent of British women in labor "reported that they had been left alone by midwives or doctors at a time when it worried them..."[299] The survey questioned some 26,000 women who delivered between January and February 2007.[300]

DAD'S CANCER UNDETECTED DESPITE 50 HOSPITAL VISITS

Imagine needing to make a hospital visit not once, not several times, but on 50 occasions. Yet, the cause for the awful pain in your stomach remains unclear.[301]

For Dunil Almeida, this situation was his own real life health care horror story. Despite being examined 50 times by various doctors, the pain in Almeida's stomach that in fact was colon cancer was somehow undiagnosed again and again under the care of the government-run British National Health Service.

This incredible tale of medical incompetence started in May 2005, when Almeida was first seen in the emergency room at London's Hillingdon Hospital. Over the next 18 months, Almeida would repeatedly return complaining of stomach pain.

But doctors failed to test for the cancer that would eventually kill him. According to Almeida's widow, Chiandra, one doctor suggested Almeida "was probably imagining the pain."

It would not be until Almeida visited Sri Lanka in January 2007 to see relatives that he learned of the cancer. He was scheduled for a long overdue abdominal scan and returned to London to see a specialist. But by the time the appointment was confirmed, it was too late. Almeida had lost over 50 pounds by this point, and, tragically, he died in February 2007, aged 42.

"I'm devastated. I feel bitter and angry," said Chiandra.

"This is an NHS disaster," charged Katherine Murphy of the Patients Association, an independent UK health care charity. "What the bloody hell was going on?"

As for Almeida's grieving wife and three children he left behind, they were given the following assurance: "A formal investigation is under way," from Susan LaBrooy, medical director of Hillingdon Hospital.

NHS TO PATIENT: COME BACK WHEN BLIND

Leslie Howard spent his life working for the British government. But that same government, which manages the National Health Service, refused to fund treatment that could save the sight of this retired Royal Military policeman and former prison officer – that is, until he went blind.

Howard, 77, from York, was diagnosed with 'wet' age-related macular degeneration (ARMD) in his right eye in November 2006. The degenerative eye condition can cause rapid vision loss,[302] and treatment is recommended immediately following diagnosis to slow its progression.[303]

Though Howard noticed his vision deteriorating by the day,[304] his local NHS provider, North Yorkshire and York Primary Care Trust (PCT), refused to provide him with potentially sight-saving drugs. It notified Howard that to be considered for a new generation of "anti-VEGF" drugs, he must first become fully blind in one eye and develop the same problem in the other eye.[305]

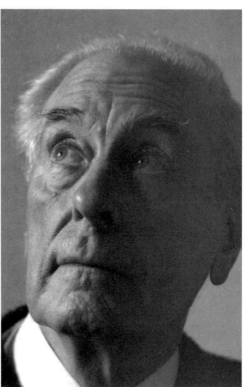

After the NHS refused to fund the drug needed to save Leslie Howard's vision, a private hospital offered him the sight-saving treatment free.

At that time, the £6,000 pound (~$9.900) a year treatment was available elsewhere in the UK under the public health care system.[306] But, seemingly, treating Howard was considered a poor value by the bean counters at his local NHS provider. "In agreement with other PCTs in the region, North Yorkshire and York PCT has agreed to fund anti-VEGF drugs for patients for whom it has been evidenced that this will be an effective treatment," said the North Yorkshire and York Primary Care Trust.[307]

"Has the government lost all sense of compassion as well as economics? Is there no way I can get help to save my sight?" a frustrated Howard asked.[308] "I can't believe I'm being left to go blind in one eye. I've spent most of my working life devoted to public service – I was in the Army, police and prison service – and I've never failed to pay my dues."[309]

For Howard and his wife, Mary Ann, purchasing thousands of pounds of private treatment was not a viable option.

"I can't afford that kind of money," Howard said. "I've paid tens of thousands of pounds in taxes and to know I'm going to lose my sight because I can't afford private treatment is diabolical. The problem is that we have lived too long and are just pieces of meat now – a nuisance."[310]

To Howard's surprise, media publicity of his dealings with the NHS prompted a private hospital to volunteer assistance. Beginning in late April 2007, as part of its 50th anniversary celebration, Nuffield Hospitals provided Howard with the first course of treatment free of charge that could save his eyesight.[311]

"When I found out that the Nuffield Hospitals had agreed to give me the treatment free of charge, there was such a feeling of elation," Howard said. "I could not quite believe it, and I cannot even begin to explain my gratitude."[312]

Howard said that a course of treatment with the drug Lucentis "stabilized and may have even improved [my eyesight] ever so slightly..."[313]

Though immensely grateful, Howard blasted the NHS for failing to help him and other wet ARMD sufferers. "I still have this feeling of immense annoyance with the PCT, not just for me, but for all the other patients who are being denied this treatment on the NHS," he said.[314]

In 2008, the National Institute for Health and Clinical Excellence, the NHS clinical standards authority, changed course to permit treatment of wet ARMD with Lucentis immediately upon diagnosis in one eye. NHS will fund the first 14 injections, and the drug's manufacturer, Novartis, will pay for additional doses.[315]

Reacting to the policy reversal, Howard said, "I am absolutely over the moon. But it is a long overdue decision, and one which will unfortunately come too late for many who have already lost their eyesight."[316]

NHS PENALIZES WOMAN FOR SUPPORTING HER OWN CANCER TREATMENT

Colette Mills of North Yorkshire, England was up against a rigid National Health Service policy that at the time would have taken away her taxpayer-provided health care if she purchased a life-extending cancer drug beyond the dosage the government provided for her.

Mills has fought breast cancer for over a quarter century.[317] Though the last roughly 20 years were "blissfully" clear of cancer, she says,[318] it returned in 2003 and spread throughout her body.[319] The 58-year-old former NHS nurse was given Taxol, a chemotherapy drug, as part of her publicly-financed health care. But, following the advice of her hospital specialist, Mills decided to spend her own money to boost her treatment with the so-called wonder drug, Avastin.[320]

Drug trials show Taxol is perhaps twice as effective when combined with Avastin,[321] and, when coupled, the drugs could slow advanced breast cancer.[322]

Mills believed that combining the drugs "would probably give me a longer life and a better quality of life."[323] She added, "Avastin may only increase your lifespan by six weeks or six months but, believe me, when it's your life, you're not picky."[324]

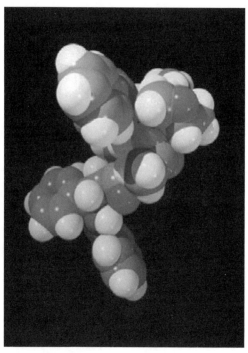

Credit: George McGregor/National Cancer Institute

After the NHS refused to provide the anti-cancer drug Taxol (molecule shown) for Collette Mills, it told her she'd lose all her NHS cancer coverage if she paid for it herself.

The rub at the time was even if Mills paid out-of-pocket to supplement her care, the NHS would begin to bill her for the entire cost of treatment because she would be considered a private patient.[325]

"If a patient chooses to go private for certain drugs they elect to become a private patient for the course of their treatment for that condition. That is trust policy," said a statement by South Tees Hospitals NHS Trust, Mills' local health care provider.[326]

Though Avastin was publicly available elsewhere in the UK,[327] South Tees Hospitals NHS Trust would not fund Avastin because of its high cost.[328] In Britain, the wide disparity of drugs and services made available depending on locality is informally termed the NHS 'postcode lottery.'

Mills was willing to pay the estimated £4,000 (~$6,600) a month to get the expensive drug and have it administered – but she did not want to be stuck with the tab for her entire treatment. "The costs would increase from £4,000 a month to about £10,000 to £15,000 for all my care. I would need to pay charges for seeing the consultant, for the nurses' time, for blood tests and scans," Mills explained.[329]

Thus, by doing what she thought necessary to improve her chances of survival, Mills would be responsible for paying some £15,000 (~$24,400) to the government. "The policy of my local NHS trust is that I must be an NHS patient or a private patient," said Mills. "If I want to pay for Avastin, I must pay for everything. It's immoral that the drugs are out there and freely available to certain people, yet they say I cannot have it."[330]

The rationale for the bizarre policy that restricted how citizens spent their own money for health care was rooted in the NHS's belief that care should be equal and not based on a patient's ability to pay. "The Government is committed to a publicly funded NHS, free at the point of use and available to all regardless of income," explained a spokesman for Britain's Department of Health. "Co-payments would risk creating a two-tier health service and be in direct contravention with the principles and values of the NHS."[331]

The health care provider, therefore, rejected Mills' request because it considered her buying an extra drug to be an "add on" to her existing NHS treatment.[332] Mills' pleas to the NHS health trust were rejected,[333] and she and husband, Eric, abandoned their challenge.[334]

"I can't go private..." said Mills. "This decision is totally unjust... this drug would prolong my life."[335]

Mills recognized there naturally may be cost prohibitions for some care. But, she argued, "The whole concept of the NHS is that it's free at the point of need. Why should that stop because I want to pay for something?"[336] She also pointed out the NHS's apparent double standard. "It is already a two-tier NHS," said Mills.[337] "I'd had a scan privately when there was a two-week wait on the NHS... If I go to the dentist I can mix my NHS and private treatment."[338]

Professor Karol Sikora, a medical expert who advises the World Health Organization, sided with Mills. "For health bosses to say Mrs. Mills cannot top up her NHS treatment is ideology gone mad. It is medical communism and utterly immoral," she charged.[339] "This is unfair to taxpayers who are entitled to NHS care. If this patient wishes to pay for another drug, that should be her choice."[340]

After considerable public disapproval and an official Department of Health Review, the NHS reversed its supplemental treatment policy in November 2008.[341] Alan Johnson, the then-Health Secretary, announced new guidelines that purchasing private treatment will not mean that patients forfeit their entitlement to NHS services.[342]

Reacting to the policy change, Mills said, "This move by the Government is exactly what I've been fighting for – but it has been a long time coming."

Although the government's change of policy was welcome news for patients like Mills, it came too late for Mills herself – four months after her unsuccessful effort to purchase Avastin herself, her cancer spread to such an extent that it will no longer respond to the treatment.[343]

HOSPITAL TURNS AWAY WOMAN IN LABOR

A pregnant Rebecca Register of North Walsham, UK awoke early in the morning in labor. But the mother-to-be would experience a delivery nightmare after she was unable to gain admittance at a government-managed hospital.

At 7:00 that morning in April 2007, Register called the Norfolk and Norwich University Hospital, a public National Health Service hospital operated by the Norfolk and Norwich University Hospital NHS Trust. Though she was near to giving birth, the hospital told Register she would have to wait for a spot to become available.[344]

"I was told to wait a bit longer," Register recalled, "despite my first child being born very quickly and having been advised not to hang about if I ever had a second child."[345]

To her horror, when Register later called a second time, she learned the public hospital's maternity ward had stopped taking in new patients. It would remain closed until 1:20 pm that day.[346]

"By this stage, I was absolutely petrified. When the person on the phone said to me that they had some bad news – the unit had just closed – my mouth just dropped open," said Register. "I was understandably very upset and frightened, which are emotions that no expectant, laboring mother should be made to feel."[347]

Midwives suggested Register drive to a different hospital some 30 miles away. Left with no choice, Register and her husband, David, frantically set out for James Paget

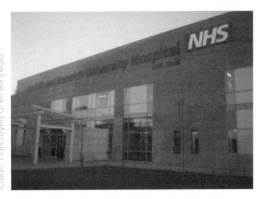

University Hospital in Gorleston. But only seven miles en route, they were forced to turn back when Register realized the hospital was too far away to get there in time. David called for paramedics, and the couple raced home.[348]

One hour later, in their living room, a midwife helped Register deliver a healthy son, Zak. The paramedics on site provided her with pain relief.[349]

Rebecca Register gave birth at home because the Norfolk and Norwich University Hospital's maternity ward was full.

"It was not my choice to have a home birth," said Register, who wanted to deliver Zak by a water birth, similar to the way she gave birth to her first child. "That was the last thing I wanted and only came about due to the shortage of midwives and care at the N&N [Norfolk and Norwich University Hospital] that day."[350]

As traumatic as her experience was, Register is not alone. On 12 occasions in 2007, the maternity ward at the Norfolk and Norwich University Hospital closed itself to new patients. Hospital managers cite a greater number of deliveries than expected as contributing to overcrowding and its inability to take in new patients.[351] The hospital did not improve its performance in 2008, a year in which the maternity unit was closed 18 times for a total of 101 hours. On one such occasion, the unit was closed for nine hours.[352]

FOUR-INCH STEP PREVENTS 98-YEAR-OLD FROM RETURNING HOME

Florrie Tranter of Sandwell, England was looking forward to getting home from the hospital. But for eight hours, hospital transportation officials kept the 98-year-old from her wish because her home's four-inch high front door step was considered a potential safety risk.[353]

After spending the evening in Birmingham's City Hospital for breathing difficulty, doctors cleared her to leave in the early morning hours the next day. But the hospital's transportation officials had other ideas. Because of the elderly woman's front door step, as a precaution, an official would investigate it before allowing Tranter to be transported.

"A transport official came round to look at the two front door steps and said they could not carry her over them because it was a safety risk," explained Tranter's son-in-law Gordon McDermott.

Carrying out one inconvenient assessment on the matter of whether paramedics could clear a four-inch step, apparently, was not enough. Hospital officials determined that a more thorough assessment was needed. But because of low staff levels, it would be several hours before this would be complete. Meanwhile, Tranter would continue to wait in the hospital.

"It [was] health and safety gone mad," described a disgusted McDermott. Appalled that hospital officials continued to strand his mother-in-law for hours and for dubious reasons, he contacted the press about the situation. This seemed to pay off. "Hours later, a second official came about the step and when I told him the local paper was getting involved, he suddenly said he would sort it out," recalled McDermott.

According to Jessamy Kinghorn, the hospital's spokesman, Tranter's eight-hour delay was "based on best practice and health and safety advice and guidance." Kinghorn continued, "Staff can have difficulty getting patients safely into their homes if a risk assessment is not carried out first."

But the family does not accept the hospital's approach. "It is absolutely appalling that my mother-in-law was taking up a bed for no medical reason and kept from her wish to go home," fumed McDermott.

NHS LEAVES CANCER SUFFERER TO FUND HER OWN TREATMENT

Barbara Moss, a former grammar school teacher from Worcester, England, was forced to use a significant chunk of her pension to save her life because the British National Health Service – to which she paid taxes to her entire working life – refused to fund a life-saving cancer drug for her when she needed it.

Doctors gave Moss, 54, up to five months to live when she was diagnosed in November 2006 with what was believed to be inoperable colon cancer, which had spread to her liver.[354] Moss was given the option of undergoing chemotherapy, but was told the NHS had no treatment that would save her life.[355] Moss was so convinced she would soon die that she began planning her own funeral and writing goodbye notes to her family.[356]

But she had newfound hope when she discovered an alternative treatment, the drug Avastin. Though this apparent 'miracle drug' offered promising results, Moss' NHS provider, Worcestershire Primary Care Trust, refused to fund the expensive treatment.[357] Worse news followed: if Moss opted to pay for the Avastin with her own money, the NHS demanded that she forgo NHS health services entirely. This would require Moss to transfer her care to a private clinic, which she would have to finance herself, paying out-of-pocket not only for the drug but also for traditional chemotherapy and services such as blood tests and oncologist appointments – all treatments she supposedly was entitled to under the NHS.[358]

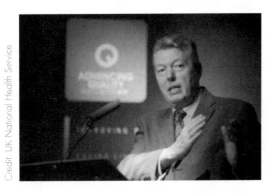

Following a public outcry, Britain's then-Health Secretary Alan Johnson announced a repeal of the policy that all Britons who pay for drugs the NHS won't cover will lose all related NHS health care coverage.

Credit: UK National Health Service

At the time, NHS policies forbade patients supplementing, or what the NHS termed 'topping up,' their care privately by paying for drugs the NHS declined to finance. No exceptions were made for life-or-death situations. NHS officials feared that allowing patients to assist in financing their own care would create a two-tiered health system.[359]

Facing death, Moss chose to take an early retirement and to use £21,000 (~$34,600) from her pension along with money from her elderly mother and her husband's pension to pay for private care at Cheltenham General Hospital.[360] "When I went in to the hospital I didn't assume I would be coming out again," said Moss.[361]

Fortunately, after four courses of Avastin alongside traditional chemotherapy, the treatment that the NHS denied her saved her life. The tumor had even shrunk enough that in October 2007, now back on the NHS, Moss underwent a five-hour operation to remove it safely.[362] Following the operation, Moss took a further course of Avastin to prevent the cancer from returning.[363]

"It was like a miracle. I had been planning my funeral – now I had life again," Moss exclaimed. "I was accepting death but now I no longer feel like I have to accept it."[364]

"This drug gave me my life back – it reduced the tumor by 50 per cent, and without it I would not be alive today," Moss firmly stated.[365]

Though thankful to have survived the cancer, Moss is upset the NHS denied her – and patients like her – the best possible care to extend her life.

"They should be ashamed of themselves – of the way they turned down the case out of hand," Moss charged. "People should be entitled to this. I would not have had my life extended without private medical health care."[366]

Moss lost her March 2008 appeal to the Worcestershire Primary Care Trust to have her Avastin treatment funded publicly as "an exceptional case."[367] But she was pleased that later that year, responding to substantial adverse publicity, the NHS reversed its co-payment ban.[368] In November 2008, Alan Johnson, then Health Secretary, announced that patients who supplement their care privately – and who must do so at a private facility – will not lose their NHS care.[369]

Curiously, while the NHS effectively abandoned Moss and patients like her, it had funds available for tattoo removals. The NHS picked up the tab to remove some 187,086 tattoos between April 2004 and March 2005, spending as much as £2,500 per procedure. One such patient, Tanya Bainbridge, formerly a sailor named Brian, made headlines in 2006 after receiving NHS funding for the removal of large "unladylike" forearm tattoos –tattoos Bainbridge reportedly wanted removed in order to enhance her appearance in sleeveless dresses. Bainbridge's £20,000 sex change operation, done in 2001, also was funded publicly by the NHS.[370]

WAR VETERAN WAITS TWO YEARS FOR HEARING AID; GIVES UP AND GOES PRIVATE

Ron Bloom of Ipswich risked his life fighting in World War II for Britain. But for over two years, the government-managed National Health Service stonewalled the elderly Royal Navy veteran's attempt to get an adequate hearing aid.[371]

Since losing a great deal of his hearing in military combat, Bloom has relied upon a hearing aid to lead a normal life. But when Bloom reached age 85, the outdated analog hearing aid he had used for 20 years no longer got the job done. So when hearing became more difficult and new digital devices became available through the NHS, Bloom visited his general practitioner, who referred him to a hearing clinic.

At Ipswich hospital, Bloom was told the wait for an upgrade to a digital hearing aid would be several months. But several months turned into half a year, which grew to over two years.

"[E]very three or four months I was getting a letter saying there would be longer delays, first six months, then nine months," Bloom recalled. "The last letter I received said the wait would be even longer – because they are prioritizing children, which I think is completely the right thing to do as they have their whole lives ahead of them."

Meanwhile, Bloom's hearing continued to deteriorate. "I was always asking people to repeat themselves and if there was more than one noise in a room I didn't have a hope of hearing anything," he explained.

After more than two years of waiting, a frustrated Bloom ended up shelling out £2,000 (~$3,200) out-of-pocket for a new device instead of waiting for the government to get around to assisting him.

What is maddening to Bloom is if he lived elsewhere in Britain, he might have received a replacement hearing aid sooner. In fact, according to government figures brought to light by the Royal National Institute for Deaf People, a London-based charity, the average wait to receive a hearing aid is 78 weeks in Bloom's county of Suffolk in the far eastern region of England – the second longest wait time in Britain.[372] By contrast, patients in western counties experience a wait of only 13 weeks. The wide discrepancy of available health services and care across localities in Britain is referred to crudely as the NHS "postcode lottery."

"I think it is disgraceful that if I lived a few miles away in Norwich I would have got my digital hearing aids within four weeks," fumed Bloom. "It makes me sick to think that if I lived almost anywhere else in the country I would have got them much quicker. I feel very badly let down after paying taxes all my life."

Some 59 hospitals in Britain have wait times longer than one year for analog-to-digital hearing aid upgrades, according to a survey by the British Society of Audiologists.[373]

PATIENT FLIES 5,000 MILES TO ESCAPE NHS WAIT

Sarah Paris of Devon, England avoided a year of waiting for treatment from the British government's 'universal' National Heath Service by flying some 5,000 miles to a private hospital in India.

In October 2003, Paris injured her shoulder while doing home repair. She got by for months on private physiotherapy, which she paid for out-of-pocket. But her condition gradually became more serious.[374]

"I couldn't drive, I couldn't sleep, [and] I was getting more and more angry with my kids, because I was in so much pain," Paris recalled.[375]

When she could not move her arm and had to put it in a sling, the former police officer went to her general practitioner in March 2004.[376] That's when Paris learned it would be a six-to-eight week wait to see a NHS physiotherapist. Moreover, for surgery, the combined wait for an assessment and the operation was close to one year.[377]

"I was told I would have to wait a year for surgery even if they booked me in for it, which they were very reluctant to do," Paris explained.[378]

Instead of waiting in pain for eventual NHS care, Paris contacted Apollo Hospital[379] – a private Indian health care corporation that owns and manages some 41 hospitals. Apollo offered immediate care "for a fraction of the price," Paris said.[380]

In one week, the hospital arranged surgery and luxury recuperation facilities to boot at a cost of £1,500 (~$2,400). Despite a £550 (~$900) flight, Paris considered going overseas a bargain.[381] An equivalent operation at a private facility in Britain would have cost her over £10,000 (~$16,000).[382]

Three days after her arrival in Chennai, India, surgeons repaired Paris' shoulder.[383] Afterward, she raved about her care. "The thing that impressed me most was how caring they were. They gave me a 24-hour nurse, who was really sweet. If I went anywhere, they'd send a driver, a security guard and a nurse – I felt a bit like a celebrity!"[384]

She continued, "Then I stayed in a spa afterwards and had a great time. It was a five-star hotel with Ayurvedic treatment [an ancient Indian practice], which was fantastic and a fraction of the price it would be here."[385]

Paris is among the tens of thousands of Britons fueling the booming health tourism industry. Traveling abroad for health care is increasingly appealing for those fed up with long NHS waits or fearful of acquiring an infection in a government hospital.[386] In fact, in 2007 an estimated 100,000 Britons had treatment in a foreign country for medical services ranging from major surgery to cosmetic work and dentistry.[387]

TERMINAL CANCER SUFFERER'S MIXED-SEX WARD MISERY

Patricia Balsom's final days fighting terminal cancer were spent in agony and frustration at a government-run mixed-sex ward in the Greater London town of Uxbridge.[388]

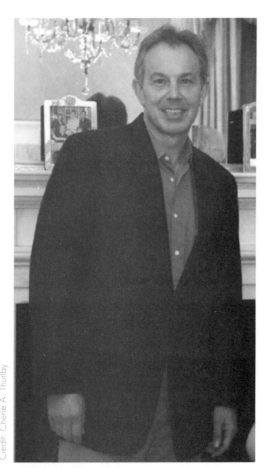

Credit: Cherie A. Thurlby

Despite explicit campaign promises, as prime minister, Tony Blair failed to abolish mixed-sex wards in NHS hospitals.

In early 2006, Balsom collapsed in her home and was taken to the hospital. She was diagnosed with lung and brain cancer.

In a diary entry, Balsom wrote, "Because of my age – 57 – I was told that very little could be done for me, and that I had up to six months left to live."

Fortunately, Balsom's sister, Janet Street-Porter, covered the £15,000 (~$24,000) necessary for Balsom to have gamma knife treatment done privately. "It was after this that the NHS offered me a course of radiotherapy on my lungs, which I had in July," wrote Balsom in her diary.

In September, an MRI scan showed the brain cancer had receded, and Balsom was offered a bone scan by the NHS. Despite pain in her ribs, Balsom had to wait at home for two weeks until the end of October to be scheduled for the vital scan, which would determine if the cancer had spread to her bones. Meanwhile, she was given an X-ray. But on the morning of the appointment, Balsom became ill and was admitted to the observation ward at Hillingdon Hospital, where she was due for the scan.

"I was seen by doctors who slightly changed my medication and told me I could go home on Monday [five days after being admitted]... I was told that a carer from an agency would come in every day and help us. No one mentioned whether I would ever get a bone scan," Balsom wrote.

In the mixed-sex ward where she was admitted, Balsom recalled being awakened twice one night by a man opposite her in their shared unit. "He was standing stark naked at the end of his bed masturbating," she wrote in disgust.

While at Hillingdon, she was given only one pillow and refused a spare to prop up her leg, as a nurse instructed, to ease the swelling caused by a blood clot. She was discharged the same day, not in an ambulance, but by taxi along with what Balsom described as a "trainee nurse" who made sure to take back an oxygen device used during the transfer.

Two days later, Balsom was back in the hospital because of breathing difficulties and again placed in the mixed-sex ward. She was given oxygen and morphine and, to her horror, asked if she wanted to be resuscitated if she collapsed, as she was terminally ill. The following day, she was discharged in the back of a NHS delivery van without a nurse and with only enough medication of one prescription to last a day.

"I feel Hillingdon Hospital are making whatever time I have left so much more stressful than it need be. They are cheating me out of quality time with people I care about. Apologies aren't enough, they don't buy time back," Balsom wrote.

The final diary entry on the day before she died read: "Up all night with pain. Crying and want to go in a nursing home to die because I cannot put my husband through all this... I don't feel as if anyone in the NHS is really in charge of my case. It's all up to me, [sister] Janet and [husband] Mick."

Balsom passed away on November 16, 2006, never having received a bone scan and, according to the diary, seen only twice by a doctor during her final two weeks. She wrote in her diary that she believed her care was rationed because she suffered from more than one form of cancer and was unlikely to recover.

"Pat's final wish was that what happened to her would never happen to anyone else who happened to live in the borough of Hillingdon," said Janet Street-Porter.[389]

The ruling British Labour government promised to abolish mixed-sex wards in its 1997 and 2001 campaign manifestos. But a 2007 report by the Healthcare Commission, formerly the independent NHS watchdog,[390] found that roughly a third of Britain's admitted emergency patients are forced to share mixed-sex hospital bathrooms and to sleep in mixed-sex accommodation units.[391]

In January 2009 – 12 years after Labour's pledge – Alan Johnson, then Health Secretary, announced a £100 million (~$162 million) initiative to convert the remaining 15 percent of NHS hospitals to single sex accommodation. Beginning in 2010, the government will fine hospitals that treat patients in mixed-sex wards.[392]

NHS TELLS DISABLED MAN WITH FIST-SIZE HERNIA TO WAIT FOR SURGERY

Tony Pople of Claydon, in the east of the United Kingdom, is severely disabled. He suffers from the genetic condition Fragile X Syndrome. Because he has severe physical and mental handicaps, Pople requires around-the-clock care from his sister, Gillian Harris, 61, and her husband, Gordon, also 61.[393]

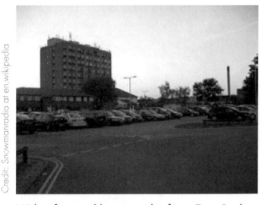

Credit: Snowmanradio at en.wikipedia

With a fist-sized hernia on his face, Tony Pople needed surgery fast – but Ipswich Hospital cancelled his surgery three times.

Pople's troubles became worse when a hernia on his face grew to the size of a fist. Luckily, his family was by his side to help when Britain's government-run National Health Service offered no sympathy.

The NHS has bragged it is "recognized as one of the best health services in the world by the World Health Organization."[394] Yet, despite Pople's need for urgent treatment, the NHS put off operating on Pople's hernia three times in six days.

In March 2007, the Ipswich Hospital cancelled Pople's surgery the day before it was to take place. As Pople's hernia advanced, his family became increasingly anxious. "I'm not a doctor but I was looking at him and just praying to God it was going to get done," said Gordon Harris. "It was a terrifying situation, he [Pople] couldn't stand up right because of it [the hernia] and at times he had been feeling sick as well."

Surgery was rescheduled twice more before it finally was carried out at the end of March. Nevertheless, the difficulty of getting Pople to and from the hospital brought his family nearly to the point of exhaustion. "You would not believe what we have to go through to get him to the hospital, a special bus has to be booked and we have to sort out our two boys who go to Genesis Orwell Mencap five days a week," said Gordon Harris.

In addition to caring for Pople, Gordon and Gillian Harris supervise their two disabled adult sons, aged 35 and 38.

The hospital apologized, but it is no consolation for the Harris family, which has made a formal complaint. "One of our difficulties is that we try to treat everyone as individuals. But sometimes we don't live up to our own high standards," said an Ipswich Hospital spokesman.

MAN ENDURES EIGHT-HOUR DELAY FOR HOSPITAL TREATMENT

Wesley White awoke during the middle of the night with a tormenting stomach pain.[395] The 63-year-old from Bellingham, England would have to wait over eight hours in agony for the government's National Health Service to get him necessary treatment in a hospital.

Two and a half hours later, Wesley's wife, Jan White, decided White's condition was serious enough to call NHS Direct, a 24-hour taxpayer-funded advice hotline staffed by nurses. Jan called back twice over the next three and a half hours before an after-hours doctor arrived at the couple's home. Because the rural town of Bellingham no longer has an after-hours doctor or even a dedicated ambulance through the NHS, the doctor sent had to travel from outside Newcastle, over 30 miles away.

"My wife rang NHS Direct at 5:30 am, but now I just wish I had dialed 999 [emergency services] straight away," White said. "The service is totally inadequate. Having an ambulance or an on-call doctor here would have made all the difference. They have cut rural ambulances and out-of-hours doctors and there is a chance that it could kill somebody."

The doctor arrived at the Whites' home at 9:45 am and determined an ambulance was needed. But it would take until 12:15 pm for it to arrive from yet another town 35 miles away. Worse yet, the paramedic crew was not equipped for urgent care and was unable to provide morphine. A second ambulance had to be called, arriving 15 minutes later.

By this point, White's condition was so severe that he needed to be airlifted to Royal Victoria Infirmary in Newcastle. At 2 pm, finally, White received hospital treatment, and three days later had his appendix removed. He was thereafter released to recover at home.

"If my appendix had burst I would have been a goner. In those situations, minutes can make a difference, let alone the hours I had to wait," he said. "I just want this to be put into the public domain for the sake of other people who might not make it, thanks to these stupid policies."

"The time it took is just unbelievable and I am very angry," White continued. "I am not a vindictive person, but I would like to see something like this happen to one of the people who make the stupid health service policies to make them see sense."

White's neighbor, Jim Brownbridge, was appalled that it took so long to get White treatment. "It is absolutely ridiculous. The local NHS is supposed to be hard up yet the cost of the services on that day must have been massive. It could have been avoided... If Bellingham still had an ambulance and doctors in surgeries out of hours, he would have been taken far earlier in the day."

One possible explanation for the long ambulance wait is that White may have been the victim of an alleged NHS practice called "patient stacking."[396] According to government records, tens of thousands of sick patients have been left to wait for hours inside an ambulance before being admitted to hospital accident and emergency departments. The alleged practice allows hospitals to better meet government health targets for admitting, transferring or discharging emergency patients within a four-hour time limit.[397]

As a consequence of "patient stacking," ambulances in use as "mobile waiting rooms"[398] cannot respond to new emergency calls.[399]

GOVERNMENT TELLS CANCER PATIENT: WE'LL TAKE AWAY YOUR HEALTH CARE IF YOU PAY FOR SUPPLEMENTAL CARE YOURSELF

Debbie Hirst of Carbis Bay, England was desperate enough to get the drugs she needed to fight terminal breast cancer that she would sell her house. Though she was in a fight for her life, the British National Health Service told Hirst that if she bought life-extending drugs – that is, legal drugs, privately, using her own money – she would no longer receive the NHS's taxpayer-financed care she was entitled to.[400]

The 57-year-old was diagnosed with cancer in 1999. She received treatment on the NHS at Christie Hospital in Manchester, but the cancer became so advanced that she was given only eight weeks to live by 2003. Hirst beat the odds, surviving for years,[401] and when the cancer spread to her liver and bones in 2007,[402] she looked for an aggressive treatment.

Hirst's doctor suggested she would "benefit massively" from taking Avastin,[403] an expensive anti-cancer drug widely used in Europe as well as the U.S.[404] Though Avastin was licensed in England, the NHS did not provide it.[405] Thus, for Hirst to get it privately, it would cost her a staggering £60,000 (~$98,000).[406]

Nevertheless, believing time was running out, Hirst began to save, having been told by her oncologist that she would be allowed to fund her own Avastin treatment.[407] She raised some £10,000 (~$16,200) by December 2007 with help from family and friends and put her home on the market.[408] That's when she got the devastating news that government rules at that time prohibited supplementing NHS care with private treatment. If she received Avastin privately, even while paying for it herself, Hirst would be billed for the *entire cost* of her NHS health care.[409]

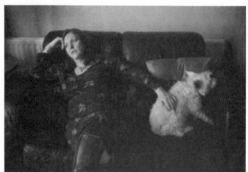

"[The doctor] looked at me and said: 'I'm so sorry, Debbie. I've had my wrists slapped from the people upstairs, and I can no longer offer you that service,'" Hirst recalled. "I said, 'Where does that leave me?' He said, 'If you pay for Avastin, you'll have to pay for everything.'"[410]

With eight weeks to live, Debbie Hirst needed the cancer drug Avastin to save her life. The NHS refused to provide it, and refused to allow her to buy it herself – although other patients were permitted to do so.

The cost of scans, hospital accommodation and so on would be hundreds of thousands of pounds,[411] making it impossible for Hirst to afford Avastin. "I was heartbroken because I thought it was cruel and rotten," Hirst said. "If I can fund it why can't they accept that money?"[412]

The rationale for the NHS's policy that banned so-called 'private co-payments' was to prevent richer patients from receiving preference over poorer ones.[413] Patients "cannot, in one episode of treatment, be treated on the NHS and then allowed, as part of the same episode and the same treatment, to pay money for more drugs," explained Alan Johnson, then-British Health Secretary. "That way lies the end of the founding principles of the NHS."[414]

But Hirst's lawyer thought the government's attempt to forbid Hirst from buying her own drugs in the name of equality was ridiculous. "The argument supporting the desire to avoid a two-tier system within the NHS is spectacularly flawed," said

Mellissa Worth. "There already exists a two-tier system arising out of the fact that some trusts [local NHS providers] sanction the use of complementary drugs like Avastin."[415]

Moreover, what further appalled Hirst was three other patients at her hospital, the Royal Cornwall Hospital, were paying for Avastin privately and able to continue their usual NHS treatment.[416] According to the New York Times' investigation, these three patients had supplemented their care before the government issued rules forbidding the practice. "Because their treatment began before the Health Department explicitly condemned the [private co-pay] practice, they have been allowed to continue," wrote the Times.[417]

Fed up that she had "been cheated out of care,"[418] as Hirst put it, she approached the news media to publicize her NHS horror story. "[I]t makes me so angry that even though I'm prepared to contribute thousands for my care they [NHS] won't even meet me halfway," she said.[419]

Hirst planned to sue the Cornwall & Isles of Scilly Primary Care Trust, her local NHS provider, over the co-payment ban.[420] But in February 2008 a review panel ruled that Hirst's condition had deteriorated sufficiently for the government to pay for her Avastin treatment, beginning on February 8.[421]

The news was "better than winning the lottery," Hirst exclaimed.[422] "It's like Christmas… My solicitor [lawyer] threatened that if we hadn't heard from the health trust responsible by 4 pm on Friday, she would begin a judicial review – and we had a call at 4 pm saying I could have the treatment on the NHS."[423]

Hirst said the legal pressure applied and media interest had something to do with the NHS changing its mind to pay for her treatment. "I would say to anyone who finds themselves in this terrible situation 'Make a fuss and keep fighting – it could save your life.'"[424]

The NHS reversed its policy banning co-payments in November 2008. Patients who pay for private treatment administered in a private facility will not lose their NHS care.[425]

UNATTENDED WOMAN IN LABOR DROWNS IN HOSPITAL BATHTUB

Midwives at a British National Health Service hospital left Lorraine Maddi unattended in a bathtub for 45 minutes while she was in labor, despite being warned that she suffered from a condition that at times caused her to faint in stressful situations.

When Maddi was discovered submerged and unconscious, doctors had to deliver the unborn baby by emergency caesarean section.[426] The baby survived, but the lack of oxygen to Maddi's brain killed her.[427]

On June 1, 2007, Maddi went into labor and was taken to Bassetlaw Hospital in Worksop, England. A family friend, Paul Guthrie, accompanied her because visa complications had prevented Maddi's foreign husband, Phaninder Maddi, from immediately flying back from India to be with her during labor.[428]

After Maddi was admitted, a midwife suggested she take a warm bath to help ease her pain.[429] When the friend stepped out to gather some of Maddi's belongings, he made sure to inform midwives that he was leaving and he reminded them to monitor Maddi

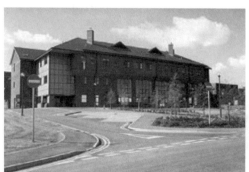

Lorraine Maddi, who suffered from a fainting disorder, was left alone in a bathtub in Bassethaw Hospital in Worksop, England.

closely, because of her history of fainting attacks. Maddi previously had written to the hospital that, because of the recent death of her mother, she had been suffering these attacks more frequently.[430]

But when Guthrie returned 45 minutes later, Maddi was still in the bathtub and the door was locked. When she did not respond to knocks, midwives opened the door to find her submerged and not breathing.[431] She had turned blue from lack of oxygen.[432]

Doctors performed emergency surgery to rescue the baby, Jayden. Though Maddi was resuscitated, she would not recover. Tragically, she died eight days later in intensive care.[433]

"My son will never know his mother," said shocked father, Phaninder Maddi.[434] "My son might not even have been alive if Paul hadn't come back when he did. I just hope that something good will come out of losing my wife."[435]

According to an investigation into Maddi's death, a midwife knocked on the door while Maddi was in the bath, but did not check further when Maddi did not reply.[436]

"A number of midwives said it was assumed she would not have been left alone during her bath, but hospital officials admitted there were no official guidelines on whether women should be left on their own," the British Telegraph reported.[437]

Since the unexpected death of his wife, Phaninder Maddi said he would take legal action to claim compensation from the Doncaster and Bassetlaw Hospitals NHS Trust,[444] which runs Bassetlaw Hospital. Meanwhile, the British government granted him residency rights, making it possible for him to raise his son in England.[439]

"She would have been a wonderful mum. I don't know what I am going to tell Jayden when he is older," said Maddi's husband. "I have this dream everyday that Lorraine's playing with Jayden and her mum is there playing with him too, saying how gorgeous he is. Then I wake up every morning and there is nothing there."[440]

AFTER MOM IS TWICE TURNED AWAY FROM OVERCROWDED HOSPITAL, FATHER DELIVERS BABY AT HOME

A Welsh father had little choice but to become a temporary doctor when the mother of his child went into labor after twice being turned away from a hospital.

Anthony Jones and his girlfriend, Elizabeth Jones, rushed to Princess of Wales Hospital early in the morning, thinking Elizabeth was going into labor. Elizabeth had been monitored at this hospital twice per week during her pregnancy because her baby was growing slowly.[441] She fully expected to deliver at the same government hospital, which is close to her home.

However, upon arrival at the hospital's maternity department, Anthony and Elizabeth were told that all the doctors were occupied with other patients and there were no beds available. Though Elizabeth was experiencing strong contractions, a midwife she spoke with did not examine her and told the couple to come back later.[442]

"They told us they were shut because they were full and to go have a cup of coffee and come back," said Anthony. "We only live five minutes up the road, so we went home."[443]

"It was one big shock," said Elizabeth. "I wanted to have her in the hospital after all the problems we had. I knew she was coming soon because the pain was strong."[444]

Three hours later, at roughly 11:30 am, Elizabeth's contractions became more frequent. Because there was not another nearby hospital, the couple returned to the packed Princess of Wales. This time a different midwife examined Elizabeth.[445] But the midwife insisted the baby's birth was "hours away,"[446] and in any event the hospital could not accommodate the delivery until 5 pm. Elizabeth was given painkilling tablets and, again, sent home.[447]

"Other women in labor were also being turned away and told to sit downstairs in the coffee shop," recalled Elizabeth. "I don't think it's right to expect women who are in a lot of pain to go and sit in a public place."[448]

Minutes after the frustrated couple returned home, Elizabeth's water broke and she went into labor.[449] Without any medic to deliver the baby, Anthony, a bus driver, was left to receive instructions by phone, which his 17-year-old eldest daughter, Kirsty, relayed.[450]

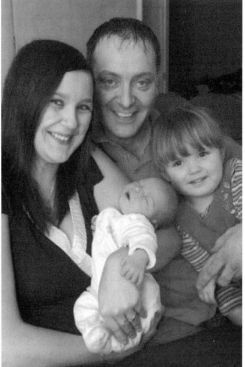

When she went into labor, Elizabeth Jones twice tried to check into the NHS's Princess of Wales hospital, but it was full. Her bus driver boyfriend delivered baby Emily at home.

"It was so quick that I didn't have time to think about it," said Anthony. "I was shocked but just had to get on with it. I was getting instructions on the phone from the 999 [emergency dispatch service] operator."[451]

Paramedics arrived to the home as the baby's head was showing. The paramedics did not take over and allowed Anthony to continue. "[T]hey said I was doing a good job and I should just carry on," he explained, as the paramedics closely looked on. "I delivered her into the world with the paramedic standing by to help me if anything had gone wrong."[452]

Thankfully, nothing did go wrong, and Anthony delivered a healthy six pound, eight ounce baby girl, Emily.[453] After the birth, two midwives came to the home to check on Elizabeth and the newborn.[454] "It was a great experience – but at the time I wished we were in hospital in a controlled environment," said Anthony. "What if something had gone wrong?"[455]

"Anthony did a fantastic job," praised Elizabeth, "but it's not what we expected from the NHS."[456] She continued, "I had no pain relief and it was agonizing. I am very unhappy about how I was treated – thankfully, the birth was straightforward."[457]

Anthony is equally upset that his girlfriend was denied care. "You hear so much about the NHS being under pressure but you would think that maternity would be a priority. Many things can wait for a later appointment — but never a baby… It's very worrying that they haven't got the facilities to do the job properly when you want it."[458]

Nationwide, UK hospital maternity wards are severely understaffed. According to a 2007 report by BLISS, a London-based charity, "Over 2,600 more neonatal nurses are needed to meet the recommended nursing level…"[459] Moreover, a national survey of 195 neonatal units found that "units in our survey were forced to refuse new admissions for an average total of two weeks in six months."[460]

SICK GRANDMOTHER WAITS 24 HOURS FOR A HOSPITAL BED

A severely ill 73-year-old grandmother waited almost 24 hours in a hospital chair before being given a bed.[461]

In January 2008, Valerie Tarr of Llanrumney, Wales, who also suffers from arthritis, came down with pneumonia. Her general practitioner believed her condition to be serious enough to warrant admission at Llandough Hospital in Penarth for treatment.

Unfortunately, the hospital did not have an available bed for her. Tarr was forced to spend the whole night in a waiting area wearing nothing more than a nightgown and robe.

"She is generally not very well," explained daughter, Jacqui Newman, at the time. "She needed to be in a bed, but the only place the nurses could find for her was this chair."

Newman and one of her children stayed with Tarr throughout the night in disbelief at the hospital's lack of care. Tarr was exhausted and unable to eat but, at last, was admitted to a bed the next day.

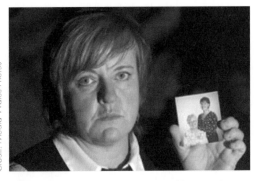

Credit: Media Wales Photos

Jacqui Newman holds a picture of her mother, Valerie Tarr, who waited for nearly 24 hours in a chair in an NHS hospital waiting for a bed to become available.

"She was in agony because of the arthritis in her neck and generally looked terrible because of the pneumonia," said Newman. "I'm not prepared to have my mother treated like this."

According to government service targets, 95 percent of new patients should spend less than four hours in an emergency department from the time of arrival to be admitted, transferred or discharged; no patient should wait longer than eight hours.[462]

According to the report produced by the Welsh Assembly Government, the four-hour target was met just 84.7 percent of the time at the Trust's major hospitals between December 2007 and December 2008.[463]

"There's no doubt the NHS is in crisis and this shows just what's happening to sick people," charged Newman.

ALL NIGHT ON A HOSPITAL GURNEY

Obtaining such basic care as a hospital bed appears to be a matter of luck for patients at one Swansea, Wales hospital. Two such patients, and a handful like them, spent all night on a hospital gurney waiting in agony when beds were unavailable – or simply closed off to them.

In October 2007, Phil Richards went to Morrison Hospital's emergency room late at night for a head injury and a possible broken nose. The government Home Office employee had fallen in his home. But instead of being treated immediately, Richards was put on a gurney to wait. Richards said he was not the only patient nurses did not offer a bed because none were available.[464]

"I, along with at least four other patients, spent the whole night in A&E [Accident and Emergency] on trollies (gurneys). I was told there were no beds available and the bed manager was aware of the situation," he said.[465]

Instead of getting needed rest, Richards was left to observe the ruckus in the hospital that night. "I was there all night and witnessed some horrific sights, mostly from blood-soaked drunken individuals who had fallen or been assaulted," he said. "From the nurse's tone it appears that this was becoming a regular occurrence."[466]

Responding to concerns about the use of such makeshift equipment, a spokesman for Swansea NHS Trust, which manages Morrison Hospital, was confident there had been improvement. "We are happy to report that since these procedures have been put in place we have seen less pressure and sufficient bed space available during busy weekend periods."[467]

Despite these assurances, the experience of another Morrison patient, Lisa Lewis, months later was similar.

Lewis, a 23-year-old student, arrived at Morrison just after midnight. She was vomiting non-stop and unable to stand. She was immediately placed on a gurney and given gas and air to relax her so that doctors could begin an examination. "[L]ittle did I know that for the next 10-and-a-half hours, this was also to be my bed," Lewis said.[468]

But the gas irritated an allergy and made Lewis sicker. She was given morphine and put on a drip because of dehydration, and doctors decided to perform an X-ray. "[A]fter overhearing staff saying something had shown up, I was relieved that at least they knew what... might be wrong and I would soon be treated... I was wrong."[469]

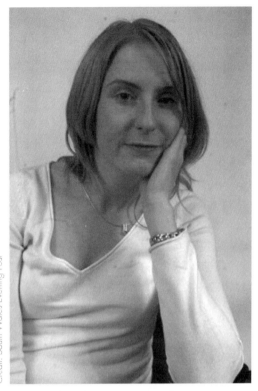

Credit: South Wales Evening Post

Suffering from kidney stones and vomiting non-stop on a Thursday, Lisa Lewis could not get a hospital bed because the hospital closes on weekends.

Doctors could not determine the cause of the ailment right away. Several hours after the X-ray, Lewis was still waiting on the gurney without answers, despite there being empty beds in the hospital.[470]

"It was too long to be waiting in a lot of pain, especially as the nurses on Ward H said there were a lot of empty beds – but they didn't want to take me out onto the ward [on a Thursday] because they close it on a weekend," explained Lewis.[471]

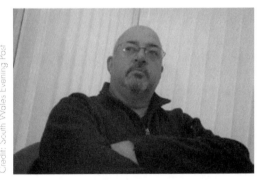

Credit: South Wales Evening Post

Phil Richards and four other patients spent a night on hospital gurneys when Morrison Hospital in Wales was full.

With Lewis waiting in a cubicle in the early morning, at last a surgeon said the X-ray revealed small kidney stones were stuck in Lewis' urinary tract. They planned to remove the stones, and hours later Lewis was told a bed had opened up in a medical admissions ward.[472]

"My delight was to be short-lived," Lewis recalled. "The porters pushed me into the much-awaited ward, where they were greeted by nurses... They said there was no bed available for me."[473]

Instead, Lewis was forced to wait in a recliner alongside other patients trying to rest without pillows or blankets.[474] Fortunately for Lewis, the next day hospital staff reopened the closed ward, and Lewis was given a bed at 11 am.[475] But by Friday – 24 hours after arriving at the hospital – Lewis had still not been operated on.[476]

"I asked a doctor when I would have my kidney stone removed," she said. "Incredibly, he told me there was no record of me having a stone and it was more likely I had a gall stone... This baffled me because I had my gall bladder removed four years ago."[477]

On Saturday, though still ill and without surgery, Lewis was discharged. She returned to the hospital two days later for morphine but received no word about whether there would be a follow up examination.[478]

"I was surprised they sent me home. I hadn't eaten since Wednesday because I was so ill all day – they said they would keep an eye on me but they just discharged me," Lewis said.[479]

THIRD TIME'S THE CHARM IN GETTING AMBULANCE FOR 81-YEAR-OLD

An elderly Scottish woman nearly died at home because emergency dispatch operators twice refused to send an ambulance to her aid, finally sending one only after three requests.[480]

81-year-old Mary MacBean of Hilton, Scotland broke her pelvis when she fell at home. The fall left McBean, who had who survived a stroke 18 months before, limp and unable to stand. Nevertheless, she managed to crawl across the floor to receive a phone call from her son, Michael, who learned of her injury.

"As soon as I realized she was hurt I raced into my car – I didn't even put my shoes on and I just drove up to her house," Michael McBean recalled.

Upon arriving, Michael found his mother "screaming in agony." While coming to her aid, Martin MacPherson, a friend called on to assist, dialed emergency services. "I was trying to hold her while Martin dialed 999 [emergency services]," Michael said.

To their amazement, an operator insisted an ambulance would not be sent immediately because Mary McBean's condition was not "life-threatening." Moreover, McBean would have to wait up to three and a half hours for an ambulance. The quickest way to get help would be to drive to the hospital, the operator told them.

"I said [to the operator] she had broken something. They said it wasn't life-threatening and would pass on the details to NHS 24. An 81-year-old who is lying on the floor with a broken pelvis is an emergency in my book," said MacPherson.

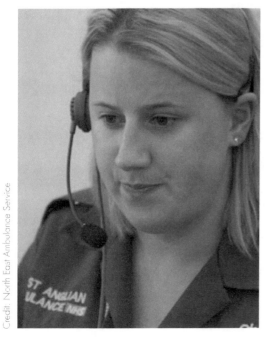

Michael McBean added, "She was being sick and sweating. Her skin was all clammy and she was beginning to drift in and out of consciousness."

At this point, Rosie Campbell, Mary McBean's daughter, arrived at the home and called emergency services. The operator again said an ambulance would not be sent immediately for a non-life threatening circumstance. Desperate, Michael McBean considered making a makeshift stretcher to transport his mother, but decided to call the emergency line himself.

Mary McBean nearly died at home because emergency dispatch operators twice refused to send an ambulance (model shown).

To his disbelief, the operator said an ambulance had been dispatched after the first call at 8:08 pm, but McBean's family and friend had not been told. "If that was the case we would not have had to call three times. Nobody mentioned this," he said. "She could have died if an ambulance hadn't come."

Twenty minutes after the third call, paramedics arrived and gave McBean morphine and oxygen. An ambulance then transported her to Raigmore Hospital, where she was successfully treated.

Following the ordeal, a Scottish Ambulance Service official justified its response policy. "We have to prioritize our resources to ensure patients with the most need are seen first. The response time of 30 minutes was appropriate in this case. Although we do appreciate Mrs. MacBean was in a lot of pain and discomfort, it was not a life-threatening situation."

ELDERLY MAN LEFT ON COLD HOSPITAL FLOOR

Staff at a government hospital in Scotland left Mitchell Cabel, 88, lying on the hospital floor for four hours after he fell. The hospital's doctors and nurses refused to move him, so paramedics were called – and they left him there for four hours.

Cabel of Ellon, Scotland had been admitted six weeks prior to Woodend Hospital in Aberdeen for treatment of a urinary tract infection.[481] But a fall from a chair immobilized Cabel on the hospital floor.[482] Instead of helping Cabel up, the nurses and doctors present left him on the floor. Nurses claimed they did not have the proper training to move the heavyset and elderly man, and said paramedics would have to be called in to lift Cabel.[483]

Roughly an hour and half after the fall, Cabel's family arrived at the hospital, shocked to find him on the floor and in pain. Cabel's wife, Elsie, and their son, Mitch, confirmed that paramedics had been called earlier to lift Cabel.[484]

"He was moaning and complaining about being sore," recalled Mitch Cabel.[485] "The doctor had made repeated calls to the ambulance service, stressing the importance of my father's situation, but nothing seemed to work… I was amazed. There was a doctor there and nurses you would assume would be trained in lifting."[486]

While waiting for the paramedics to arrive, nurses wrapped Cabel in blankets, gave him morphine to dull the pain and eventually, three hours on, moved him from the cold hospital floor onto a mattress.[487] "It's incredible that in a hospital a patient is left lying on a floor and we've got to wait for paramedics to come in," Mitch exclaimed.[488]

Because Cabel's condition was not considered life threatening, he was not given priority by the ambulance workers. "Had this gentleman not been in a hospital he would have received a very much faster response," said a Scottish Ambulance Service spokesman. "The patient was suffering from a non-life-threatening injury in a hospital environment with medical staff in attendance. We have to prioritize our resources to those that need us most, which is patients in life-threatening situations."[489]

A Scottish Ambulance Service "insider" echoed this reasoning. "A patient who is already in a hospital environment with medical staff in attendance is unlikely to ever be a high priority."[490]

It would take four hours after Cabel fell for paramedics to arrive to lift him and to be taken for X-rays.[491] It was discovered that Cabel suffered no serious injuries.[492]

Afterward, National Health Service-Grampian chief executive Richard Carey explained that hospital staff were concerned about injuring Cabel. "The nurses and doctors on duty were concerned that if they moved the patient, and because of the way he had fallen, he could have suffered a fractured neck or femur."[493]

A spokesman for the Scottish Ambulance Service added:

> We were asked by a doctor at the hospital to send an ambulance within four hours. Our procedures are such that when a doctor is with a patient he will give us advice on the appropriate response. Given the situation was in a hospital attended by medical staff and the patient didn't have a life-threatening condition, our procedures were all followed appropriately.[494]

But Mitch challenges the health authorities' explanations and questions why the hospital did not have trained staff on hand to aid his father. Mitch said:

> I later went to see a nursing manager and told her I couldn't believe that in a hospital dealing with the elderly there hadn't been a fall before... She told me my father had had a different type of fall, which I found totally unbelievable... The whole situation was unforgivable and they made it worse by trying to get me to believe their ridiculous explanations... Why was no one there with the training to lift him right away?[495]

Cabel passed away two weeks after the fall. Though it is not clear his death from kidney and heart failure related to the ordeal, what is certain is that Cabel never recovered. "I can't say that what happened to him contributed to his death, but having kidney problems and lying on a cold floor for as long as he did hadn't helped," Mitch Cabel said.[496]

AMBULANCE REFUSES TO TAKE WHEELCHAIR-BOUND EIGHT-YEAR-OLD HOME

Eight-year-old Kerry Liddle suffers from the neurological disorder cerebral palsy. The severely-disabled youngster from Tayport, Scotland was in a full body cast following hip surgery and required the use of a specially-equipped wheelchair to be mobile. The government National Health Service (NHS Scotland) left Kerry to wait six hours for an ambulance because of a shortage of vehicles – only to then refuse her a ride because she needed her wheelchair.[497]

Kerry and her mother, Lynne, were taken by ambulance to Ninewells Hospital for treatment to clear up sores under the body cast. Treatment was complete within an hour, and Kerry, confined to her wheelchair, was cleared to be transferred back home.

But four hours later, Kerry and her mother were still waiting for the ambulance. The waiting area where Kerry was placed closed. Staff then transferred Kerry to another waiting room in the hospital's child-care wing. Yet another two hours of waiting passed. Finally, an ambulance arrived, only to refuse to take both Kerry *and* the wheelchair.

"I was furious," said Lynne. "They said they could take us home but not the wheelchair, but I told them absolutely not. It would be like leaving Kerry's own legs behind."

The ambulance crew claimed the ambulance could not accommodate the girl's specially-equipped wheelchair. But, curiously, the wheelchair was not an issue on the initial transfer to the hospital: "I can't understand why an ambulance was able to take us to Ninewells [hospital], including the wheelchair, and not take us home again," said Lynne.

Though the ambulance's refusal to transfer Kerry infuriated hospital nurses, there was little they could do but call for a taxi. Kerry and her mom were allowed to charge the fare for the taxi ride back home to the hospital but not before spending six hours waiting at the hospital.

Following the ordeal, a spokesman for the Scottish Ambulance Service offered this explanation: "While this child's injuries were clearly uncomfortable and upsetting for the family, they were not life threatening… It would not be wise to remove an emergency vehicle from rotation for the duration of the trip from Ninewells to Tayport until all of the more serious calls had been dealt with." He added: "However, what is not clear is why the ambulance refused to take the child home without her wheelchair."

A spokesman for the NHS admitted, "To wait six hours for an ambulance, only to be told when it turns up that it can't accommodate a wheelchair, is really unacceptable."

CANADIAN TOLD TO WAIT 4½ MONTHS TO LEARN IF BRAIN TUMOR IS MALIGNANT

Imagine you are told you have a brain tumor. Further imagine your wait to test if your tumor is cancerous or merely benign will be over four months.

This is the very real situation Canadian Lindsay McCreith faced in Canada's public system of "universal" – yet rationed – medical care.

McCreith, a 66-year old resident of Newmarket, Ontario, suffered a stroke in January 2006. Doctors at the Southlake Regional Health Centre in Newmarket told McCreith a CT scan showed he likely had a malignant brain tumor, but they would not be certain until a MRI diagnosis confirmed the tumor's severity – and that the waiting list for an MRI would be four and a half months long.[1] Because Canada's health monopoly forbids citizens from holding private care insurance and doctors from accepting private payment for treatment,[2] there was little McCreith could do legally in Canada but wait.

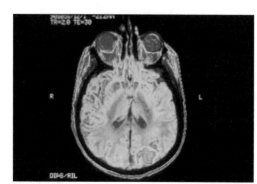

"How many people are out there getting the same kind of shabby treatment?" asked McCreith.[3]

Not willing to accept an unknown prognosis that perhaps threatened his life, McCreith's family found him a hospital across the border in Buffalo, NY that would perform an MRI scan the very next week. In Buffalo, doctors confirmed that McCreith's brain tumor was malignant. Yet, to receive treatment back in

Told he had a brain tumor, Lindsay McCreith faced a 4 ½ month wait for an MRI to find out if it was cancer.

Canada, despite McCreith's need for timely surgery, McCreith would have to wait eight months, during which time the growth could spread and become deadly.[4]

"The system stinks," exclaims McCreith. "I don't understand why there isn't a rush on government, why people say, 'I'll wait a year for a hip replacement, a year and a half to find out what's wrong with my brain.'"[5]

Fortunately, McCreith did not have to wait idly while his life hung in the balance. McCreith elected for the Buffalo hospital to remove his tumor in March 2006. Though the cost of treatment, accommodation and travel was $40,000 CAD (~$36,900), McCreith's wife, Sandra, is thankful. "We were lucky," she says. "We had that money from an inheritance just six months before from my father, so we didn't have to mortgage anything."[6]

"Had he trusted Ontario's government health care monopoly to treat him, Lindsay McCreith would likely be dead today," ran an editorial in Canada's National Post. "At the very least, his health would have been permanently diminished."[7]

McCreith is currently pursuing a lawsuit that, if successful, would permit Ontario citizens the right to pay out-of-pocket for care and to hold private medical insurance. "Citizens have a right to access health care outside the government monopoly system," says John Carpay of the Canadian Constitution Foundation, which is helping to sponsor McCreith's lawsuit.[8] In a landmark ruling in 2005, Canada's Supreme Court invalidated a provisional law in Quebec that forbid citizens there from paying privately for some procedures available under the public system.[9] However, because the case hinged on Quebec's provisional law, not national law, it is unclear whether the ruling will apply in Ontario.

IN CANADA, "FREE" CARE IS NICE – IF YOU CAN GET IT

Rev. Harry Lehotsky, a Baptist pastor and founder of New Life Ministries in Winnipeg, Canada, had a passion for aiding the poor. For over two decades, Lehotsky bettered Winnipeg's run-down inner city neighborhoods, handing out food, helping struggling residents find employment and renovating abandoned buildings for the city's impoverished residents.[10]

Lehotsky received wide praise for his work. "You'd have to look pretty hard to find anyone in Winnipeg who has made as much of a difference to their neighborhood as Harry did to his," said John Gleeson, editorial page director of the Winnipeg Sun.[11] Winnipeg Mayor Sam Katz echoed the sentiment, "He showed me and everybody else that one person can make a big difference."[12]

However, since late 2006, New Life Ministries has been without Lehotsky's leadership. Tragically, in November 2006, Lehotsky died of pancreatic cancer in his liver and spleen – cancer doctors determined was inoperable.[13]

In April 2006, Lehotsky began experiencing constant abdominal pain. Because the pain had progressed over several months, he sought an examination, but he was told it would be "months" before his family physician would be available. The second option, at the Manitoba Urgent Care Centre, was not more promising: a possible 12-hour wait in an emergency room with only one physician on duty and 20 patients ahead of him in line. Lehotsky said at the time, "I thought I'll wait until I can be treated a little more like an urgent case."[14]

Yet, the pain was so intense that Lehotsky returned to Urgent Care on Easter Sunday. "[T]hat evening the pain increased to the point I couldn't stay at home any longer. My family got me to the hospital," said Lehotsky.[15]

After Lehotsky spent a total of six hours in the emergency center, doctors were unable to diagnose a definitive ailment. Lehotsky would need to see a gastroenterologist and to make an appointment for a barium X-ray. The earliest appointment time for the X-ray was September – five months away – and November to see a gastroenterologist.[16]

"Whatever it [the ailment] was would certainly have gotten much worse – perhaps even inoperable by that point," said Lehotsky soon after. "The prospect of waiting in pain didn't excite me."[17]

Not being able to stand long or have steady meals because of the pain, Lehotsky saw yet another doctor, who prescribed a proton pump inhibitor not covered under Lehotsky's insurance.[18]

"Friends and family started finding out about my situation," Lehotsky recalled. "Responses mirrored my own feelings – everything from shock to disgust that I was paying for medical care not available to me."[19]

At long last, in May 2006, doctors diagnosed Lehotsky's condition: advanced terminal pancreatic cancer.[20] By this point, there was little medicine could do to reverse the cancer, and Lehotsky was given six weeks to nine months to live.[21]

"Surgeons have told me that there is no chance they can operate to remove something that's already spread so far inside me," Lehotsky reported to friends after this diagnosis. "Even a simple pain reduction operation to kill some of the nerves in my abdomen would likely be obstructed by the tumor."[22]

Though Lehotsky's fight against cancer ended in November 2006, his legacy is remembered in the community he worked tirelessly to improve. Colleague Trudy Turner said, "He's had a huge impact, and got the ball rolling on a lot of things and we can't afford to drop the ball now. It would be a real disservice to Harry."[23]

In February 2007, Lehotsky was appointed as a member of the Order of Canada for his life's service. This honor is considered Canada's highest achievement award.[24]

WOMAN WITH THREE CLOGGED ARTERIES DIES AFTER WAITING THREE YEARS FOR HEART SURGERY

What warrants emergency health treatment in Canada? For 58-year old Diane Gorsuch from Winnipeg, one completely clogged main artery to the heart and two other severely clogged main arteries did not cut it.

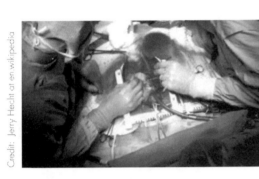

Credit: Jerry Hecht at en.wikipedia

Diane Gorsuch was on a waiting list for three years for surgery to correct a completely blocked heart artery and two partially-blocked arteries. The very day she was to have her long-awaited operation, she had a heart attack and died (model shown).

Tragically, in February 2003, Gorsuch died of a heart attack on the very day she was scheduled for cardiac surgery.[25] According to her cardiologist, the surgery would have saved her life.[26] Though Gorsuch had been waiting since 2000 for open heart surgery, doctors had bumped Gorsuch's scheduled operation twice to treat other patients with emergency cases.[27]

"This tragedy could have been avoided," said Gorsuch's son, Sean Gorsuch.[28] "My mother trusted the system with her life, it failed her."[29]

"A lot of people have died under this government's watch, and they need to be held accountable," said Sean Gorsuch. "Of course it's going to happen [again], it's only a matter of time."[30]

Unfortunately, Sean Gorsuch's remarks are accurate. According to Canada's Winnipeg Sun, between 1999 and 2003 alone,12 patients died in the Gorsuch's province of Manitoba because the medical system failed to provide timely heart surgery.[31] In 2003, there were 115 patients in Manitoba awaiting cardiac surgery.[32]

Yet, Dave Chomiak, at the time the provisional Health Minister, failed to see a systematic problem in the province's cardiac care. "In Manitoba, we do 1,200 cardiac surgeries a year. In some cases people die on the operating table. Unfortunately in some cases, people, as we found out, don't quite make it even though we have a pretty good ratio."[33]

CANADA'S REFUSAL TO FIX HOLE-IN-HEAD A REAL LIFE 'HUMPTY-DUMPTY GONE WRONG,' SAYS MEMBER OF PARLIAMENT

David Malleau of Hamilton, Ontario waited over a year for surgery literally to fix a hole in his head.

In November 2004, Malleau, then 44, was in a car accident that paralyzed one side of his body.[34] Doctors at Hamilton General Hospital removed a part of his skull the size of a fist to allow Malleau's brain enough room to swell. Malleau would need surgery to replace the missing part of his skull once the swelling decreased.[35]

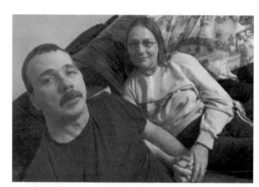

But follow-up surgery scheduled for late March 2005 was bumped because Malleau's neurosurgeon, Dr. Naresh Murty, was limited to 10 hours of work per week.[36] Instead of performing the 30-minute procedure, which also requires a two-to-three day stay in the hospital, doctors sent Malleau home and put him on a waiting list at the Hamilton Health Sciences Centre.[37]

Hamilton General Hospital left David Malleau (pictured with his wife, Pat) with a hole in his head for over a year.

For nearly a year, Malleau was a virtual prisoner in his own home, not wanting to leave or to begin rehabilitation for fear that a bump to the head would be fatal.[38] "Every month I kept calling [to schedule an operation],"[39] recalled wife Pat, who quit her job to care for her husband.[40] In Canada, "[p]ets…get better care than human beings," she added.[41]

But the Malleaus were unable to secure a new date for surgery and did not get a suitable explanation for the delay. Frustrated, they enlisted the help of Andrea Horwath, the local representative in the provincial parliament.[42]

"It was the most disgusting display of lack of responsiveness of a hospital that I've seen in a long time," said Horwath.[43] "Currently, he cannot work and has no prospect of employment or income until after this vital surgery happens. Only then can he and his family begin to rebuild."[44]

After Horwath helped publicize Malleau's situation and poor treatment by Canada's universal health service, doctors at last repaired Malleau's fractured head on January 27, 2006.[45]

"Why should it take me and our local media to get on the bandwagon and embarrass the hospital and government into doing what anybody would expect as a required procedure?," asked Horwath.[46] "When a man can't get 30 minutes of surgical time more than a year after brain surgery, we've got a big problem," she added.[47] "His life was on hold for a year because they couldn't find the time to put his skull together. It was Humpty-Dumpty gone wrong."[48]

IN ALL OF CANADA, NO SPACE FOR QUADRUPLETS

Giving birth to four identical quadruplets is as rare as winning the lottery – one in 13 million.[49] But for Canadian Karen Jepp, 35, the odds of finding an available hospital in Calgary to handle her remarkable pregnancy were just as overwhelming.

On August 10, 2007, after a little over 31 weeks carrying the four identical sisters, Jepp began to experience contractions while staying at Calgary's Foothills Medical Centre.[50] Though the infants were still two months premature, Jepp had prearranged for doctors there to monitor and to deliver her babies.[51] Yet, because of three premature births the night before, the hospital's neonatal unit was over its 16-bed capacity and therefore unable to accommodate four additional newborns.[52]

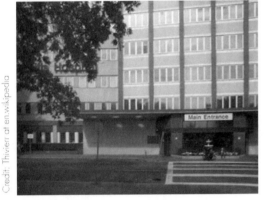

Calgary's Foothills Medical Centre (pictured) was not the only hospital unable to handle the birth of Karen Jepp's identical quadruplets – not a single hospital in all of Canada could.

Doctors had to move Jepp quickly to a different hospital. "We did an ultrasound, so we knew the babies were getting into position to be born. Her body had started her natural labor. We knew, for the health of those babies, this needed to be done," said Lynda Phelan, a spokesperson for the publicly-funded Calgary Health Region.[53]

But a search revealed there was not a Level 3 neonatal unit in all of Canada available for four premature babies together.[54] "There wasn't space anywhere in Canada, so we had to turn to our friends in Montana," Phelan said.[55] J.P., the father of the quadruplets, added, "The CHR [Calgary Health Region] had phoned clear across the country looking for beds. There were only three [neonatal intensive care] beds available anywhere in the country and they would have been in different centers across the country. That was a worse case scenario."[56]

In desperation, that evening, Karen, J.P., a nurse and a respiratory technician left Calgary by airplane for the closest U.S. hospital that reported availability – Benefits Hospital in Great Falls, Montana, over 300 miles away. On August 12, Karen Jepp gave birth to Autumn, Brooke, Calissa and Dahlia by caesarean section.[57]

"[I]t was the right decision to, to send us where... the resources were at that moment in time," said J.P. "The... staff at the Benefits Healthcare Hospital in Great Falls, Montana, were... absolutely amazing. Took care of us medically and then took care of us as people and it turns out to be a blessing in disguise that we made the trip down there and we thank them for... all their help."[58]

"It was a little disappointing they couldn't stay in Calgary where their friends and families are, but they got excellent care in Montana," said Katie, Karen Jepp's younger sister.[59] "It's frustrating. Imagine you're having quadruplets and all of a sudden you get sent away from all your friends and family."[60]

SORRY, NO BEDS FOR WOMAN IN LABOR

For Brandon Cornthwaite and his pregnant wife, Debrah, their last expectation was that a hospital would not be equipped to deliver their twin babies.

On May 27, 2004, Debrah Cornthwaite, then 27, began to experience contractions. Though she was not due to enter full-term pregnancy for another five weeks, she arrived that afternoon at her local maternity hospital, Langley Memorial, in British Columbia, Canada, in full labor.[61]

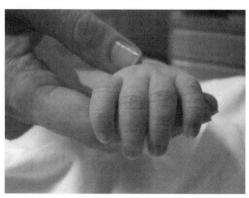

But to the couple's amazement, the hospital lacked both available beds and the expertise to handle the emergency delivery. Worse, B.C. Bedline, the province's health facility registry, was unable to locate any hospital in all of British Columbia that could accommodate the couple's soon-to-be delivered twins.[62]

When Debrah Cornthwaite went into labor, she discovered there was no hospital in all of British Columbia that could accommodate her soon-to-be delivered twins (models shown).

"You might expect this from a Third World country or if you are living out in the boonies somewhere but when you live next door to a major city... I can't believe they have no beds for two babies. I can't fathom that," Brandon Cornthwaite said.[63]

Meanwhile, Debrah Cornthwaite's contractions increased to four minutes apart. Without an available facility nearby to admit her, hospital staff looked for an alternative. "It was seven hours for the bureaucracy to get sorted out. That's unacceptable," said Brandon.[64] "Don't play with people's lives."[65]

To deliver the twins, the hospital decided Debrah would need to move to a different hospital two hours away by plane in Edmonton, Alberta. Having little choice, Debrah, Brandon and two medics boarded a chartered medical flight to Edmonton,[66] roughly 700 miles away.

During the flight, Debrah's contractions steadily increased. "We were an hour away from Edmonton and my wife's contractions got to a minute apart and thirty seconds long," Brandon said. "There was major, major concern about that… We were just praying. The medics were… just trying to hold those babies in."[67]

Fortunately, they arrived safely at Edmonton's Royal Alexandria Hospital at 11 pm, and in the early morning, Debrah gave birth by emergency Caesarean section to twin boys, Kai and Mason.[68]

"I just hope that something good can come from this and they'll do something with this health system, manage the money properly and get the qualified people, because I'm sure I'm not the first person this has happened to and I doubt I'll be the last," said Brandon.[69]

CHILD WITH CANCER PUT ON TWO-AND-A-HALF-YEAR WAITING LIST FOR MRI SCAN

Thanks to cancer, four-year-old Ryan Oldford of St. Phillip's, Newfoundland, Canada was without one of his kidneys.[70] To be certain the cancer had not spread, the Oldford family and doctors wanted an MRI examination of the boy's other kidney. Unfortunately, they faced a two-and-a-half year wait for a scan.[71]

In June 2003, Ryan lost a kidney to Wilms' tumor,[72] which is "a rare kidney cancer that primarily affects children," according to the Mayo Clinic in Rochester, Minnesota.[73] By January 2005, Ryan was considered cancer-free.[74] However, the boy's geneticist requested further screening because Ryan was at increased risk of developing leukemia as well as liver and kidney cancers.[75]

After several months of waiting,[76] the Oldfords were told the startling news: there was a two-and-a-half year wait to undergo an MRI. At the time, Newfoundland had only a single MRI machine.[77] As a result, the average wait for a scan was 30 months for children in that province – nearly double the 16-month average across Canada.[78]

"I don't think anyone at all would tell you it's reasonable for anyone to wait for an MRI for two to two and a half years – much less a cancer patient who is four years old," said Brenda Oldford, Ryan's mother.[79]

"Two years and a half is access denied," charged Normand Laberge, CEO of the Canadian Association of Radiologists. "That's just not acceptable. There's no guidelines in the world that would say that this is proper in terms of health care."[80]

What also explains the astonishing delay is Canadian children face longer wait times than adults for an MRI. "You would think kids get a priority," said Geoffrey Higgins, clinical chief of diagnostic imaging at the Health Care Corporation of St. John's. "[But] kids have to wait longer than adults. They have to wait longer [for MRI scans] than anybody else because of the sedation that's needed," he explained.[81]

Paying out-of-pocket within Canada was not an option because circumventing the publicly-financed health system for services it provides was illegal in most parts of Canada.[82] Moreover, the Canadian Association of Radiologists informed Brenda Oldford that no private clinic existed in Canada with the same level of care as a hospital.[83]

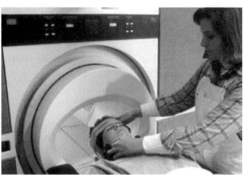

Credit: National Cancer Institute

"I felt let down by Newfoundland, and then I felt let down by Canada," said Oldford. "Canada's health care system is the envy of the world, but once you are inside, you see how individual situations work."[84]

The family had few options left. Fortunately, once Ryan's story became widely publicized, offers came in from people willing to give up their MRI appointment or to pay for Ryan's care abroad. Oldford considered taking her son to the U.S., but, fortunately, ultimately this was not necessary.[85] When one patient cancelled an MRI and another was a no-show, Ryan effectively

MRI scanners are widespread in the U.S., as shown here, but when 4 ½-year-old Ryan Oldfield of Newfoundland, Canada needed one to determine if his cancer had spread, his parents were told there would be a 2 ½-year wait.

moved to the front of the waiting list. He underwent a scan on February 2, 2005 and was determined to be healthy.[86]

Since 2005, the Canadian province of Newfoundland and Labrador has added three additional MRI machines.[87] Four machines serve a population of slightly more than half a million residents.[88]

INSIDE CANADIAN HOSPITAL, NO FOOD WHILE YOU WAIT

Betty Perras' 94-year-old mother was left to go hungry for four days while she waited for hip surgery at a Canadian hospital.[89]

In July 2007, the elderly woman (whose name has not been disclosed) checked into Rosthern Hospital in Saskatchewan, suffering from a minor stroke. While recuperating, she fell, broke her right hip and was transferred to nearby Royal University Hospital for emergency surgery.

Because of her age, it appeared that Perras' mother would be given immediate

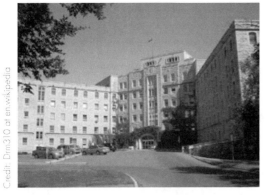

Credit: Drm310 at en.wikipedia

A 94-year-old woman was not permitted to eat on the day of her surgery – and Royal University Hospital in Saskatchewan (pictured) scheduled her for surgery four days in a row.

attention. The day she arrived at Royal University, in expectation of surgery later in the day, hospital staff provided little food.

"And then we waited," said Perras. "And we waited. And we waited some more."

During the wait, hospital workers would not provide food or drink until after 10 pm, as they were unable to predict when surgery would be scheduled, and it is dangerous for patients to eat before surgery. Unfortunately, because of painkillers, Perras' mother was unable to eat much after 10 pm. She began to lose significant weight.

"I think she should have been higher on their priority list because of her age and her condition," Perras said. "Every time they tried to move her she just about screamed."

The fourth day after Perras' mother's arrival at Royal University, surgeons replaced the ball in the broken hip joint. Surgery was successful, but Perras remained concerned that her 116-pound mother lost 12 pounds while in the hospital. She has since moved into an long-term assisted living center.

Dr. Jeff McKerrell, an orthopedic surgeon who heads the Saskatoon Health Region's orthopedic surgery, said the average wait for replacing an elderly patient's broken hip is one to two days. "She waited a little bit – longer than we would like people to wait – but not a medically unacceptable time," he said.

Perras is not pleased with the care her vulnerable mother received. "I don't think that's any way to treat our elderly people," she said. "They should have some means of opening more ORs so they can speed the process up."

Long wait times for surgery are common in Saskatchewan. A 2007 study by the Canadian-based Fraser Institute found that these residents wait an average of 27.2 weeks for surgical treatments from the time of referral by a family doctor – at the time, the longest wait in any Canadian province.[90]

SENIOR CITIZEN ABANDONS CANADA, RECEIVES LIFESAVING SURGERY IN U.S.

Shirley Healey suffered from mesenteric ischemia, a disorder that badly clogged four of her arteries. Facing probable death, the 71-year-old Canadian retiree from Vernon, British Columbia sought care from her country's so-called universal health care system but was bumped twice from scheduled surgery – apparently because of the more pressing needs of other patients.[91]

In the fall of 2005, Healey began to experience nausea, vomiting and diarrhea. She consulted her family physician, who instructed her to discontinue rheumatoid arthritis medication. But the symptoms continued, and Healey was so dehydrated that twice she went to the emergency room in the summer of 2006.[92]

A CT scan performed in a Vernon hospital revealed artery blockages in the stomach and intestine. Because the condition requires immediate treatment, Healey was booked for surgery in a Kelowna hospital roughly 30 miles from her home. But after four months went by[93] and two "urgent" appointments were cancelled (September 25 and October 6),[94] Healey said her doctor "suggested that I cross the border [into the U.S.] and get the surgery done immediately."[95]

"Anyone with blocked arteries is not meant to wait six months to a year," said Healey's doctor in Canada, Dr. Robert Ellett. "I suggested that with the way things are in Canada, I would go to the States as well."[96]

Without a guarantee another surgery would go ahead without a scheduling complication, Healey contacted a Vancouver firm, Timely Medical Alternatives, that links American hospitals to Canadian patients unable or unwilling to wait for the Canadian health care system to treat them. Healy consulted a Bellingham, Washington doctor, and the following day underwent an angioplasty stenting operation, during which a stent was inserted into four of her arteries to restore circulation. She spent one night recuperating at St. Joseph Hospital in Bellingham and returned to Canada the next day.[97]

The lifesaving surgery cost Healey some $41,000 out-of-pocket because she did not receive prior approval for it to be covered under Canada's government managed health system. But for Healey the alternative was waiting in Canada for health authorities to process paperwork while her condition deteriorated. She had lost nearly 50 pounds in one year because of vomiting and diarrhea,[98] and at the time of surgery her mesenteric artery was 99 percent shut.[99]

"If you figure you are not going to make it, then you've got to find the money," Healey said. "It's not the fault of the doctors here [in Canada], it's the health care system. It's sad that people have to pay to get their operations; but if I didn't, I wouldn't be here talking to you right now."[100]

After recovering, Healey filed an application to be reimbursed for the medical costs she undertook in America, but the provincial government in British Columbia denied her request in September 2007.[101] Healey explained, "At the moment they are saying my surgery does not qualify because it was 'elective surgery.'"[102]

As a result, Healey had been preparing a lawsuit against the British Columbia Ministry of Health seeking reimbursement.[104] With the aid of Richard Baker, founder of Timely Medical Alternatives,[104] the lawsuit was to challenge the core of the Canada Health Act, which bans private insurance.[105] Sadly, before the lawsuit was filed, Healey passed away suddenly in May 2008 from a condition "unrelated to the original complaint when she went down to Bellingham," according to Baker.[106]

"The money she spent going to the States gave her two more years of life, which she obviously lived to the fullest," added Baker. "The day she died she had just come back from playing golf."[107]

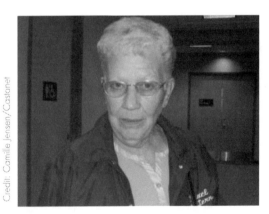

Bumped twice for urgent surgery on four clogged arteries, Shirley Healy fled to the United States for next-day treatment.

BED SHORTAGE IN CANADA STRANDS PATIENT IN U.S. HOSPITAL

Canadian Arlene Meeks' vacation received an unlikely extension when, after she underwent emergency surgery in California, she was unable to return home to Canada because of a hospital bed shortage.

In December 2007, Meeks and her husband, Wilf, of British Columbia were finishing an extended stay in Indio, California when she became ill. Though suspecting only a flu bug, Meeks learned the situation was far more serious after two local hospital visits. She needed immediate surgery to repair a ruptured appendix and to remove her gallbladder, which had become infected and gangrenous.[108]

American surgeons successfully performed an emergency operation on December 17. Yet Meeks could not be transferred back home to Canada and found herself stranded in a foreign country's hospital because there was no suitable intensive care bed available for her recovery in British Columbia.[109]

"She's frustrated as hell; she'd like to get home," said daughter Kim Meeks at the time. "She's been ready to be transported for two weeks but supposedly there are no beds for her."[110]

The health authority in British Columbia, the South Fraser Health Region, told the family there was not enough staff or available beds to accommodate Meeks at home. Moreover, if a bed did become available, there was no guarantee Meeks would not be bumped in favor of another critical patient.[111]

"They've been saying every day 'maybe tomorrow,'" complained Kim Meeks. "Basically they're just keeping her comfortable at this point; there's nothing more they can do for her. She just looks so depressed."[112]

At last, almost immediately after her experience of being stranded in California was publicized, Meeks was flown to the intensive care department at Royal Columbian Hospital in British Columbia on January 2.

Fortunately for Meeks, she and her husband took out private health insurance before leaving Canada, so it covered the costs of extended care in the U.S. and the flight home.[113]

FIVE HOSPITALS TURN AWAY APPENDICITIS PATIENT

Canadian Dany Bureau was forced to wait over a day to have an impending burst appendix removed after five hospitals turned away the 21-year-old from Gatineau, Quebec.[114] He eventually was treated following a harrowing 120-mile ambulance ride to Montreal, in which paramedics got lost en route and initially went to the wrong hospital.

At first Bureau figured his stomachache was merely indigestion. However, when the ache continued the following afternoon, Bureau and his mother decided to get his stomach examined.

A doctor at Gatineau Memorial Hospital diagnosed Bureau with appendicitis, but Gatineau Memorial could not perform the surgery. To find a surgeon, Bureau's doctor made calls to five nearby hospitals, but none could treat his patient.

"I kept getting calls saying, 'We tried Hull [Hospital], not working. Gatineau, not working. Buckingham, not working. Ottawa, not working. Maniwaki, no response.' I thought, oh my God, where are we going to end up, the States?" recalled Bureau's father, Robert Bureau.[115]

At last, an available surgeon was found – in Montreal, over 120 miles away. Not having another option and in pain, Bureau was put into an ambulance at approximately 8:37 pm to embark on the several-hour journey. Unfortunately, his ordeal was just beginning.

First, the driver could not find the correct way to the hospital. "I could hear them [the paramedics] asking directions to people outside because they didn't know where they were," Bureau said. Next, the paramedics mistakenly unloaded Bureau at the wrong hospital. At last the right hospital was found, and at 12:15 am Bureau arrived at Montreal General Hospital. His father, who had left at nearly the same time as the ambulance, had arrived 90 minutes earlier.

By this point, the surgeon, who had to wait longer than expected for Bureau to arrive, was occupied with another trauma patient. Bureau was left to wait, and would not be operated on until the next night – over 21 hours later.

"When they opened him up, it was busted. There was pus all over the place. There was dead tissue. So they cleaned it all up and they removed the appendix," Robert Bureau said.

Dany would need to stay at the hospital another four days because he developed peritonitis, a bacterial infection that, without treatment, can be life-threatening.

"As a parent, I cannot believe that there is no emergency services or surgery for our area or the Ottawa area to deal with something as simple as an appendix," said Robert Bureau.

Dany asked, "If someone had something a lot more serious than me, what would they do? Or if the Montreal hospital had no personnel, what would I have done? Where would I have gone?"

The delays could have cost Dany Bureau his life. According to a British Medical Journal Group publication, "About 17 in 1,000 people die if their appendix bursts before they have surgery."[116]

CANADIAN HOSPITAL "MESSING WITH MY DAUGHTER'S LIFE"

Julia de Zeeuw, a 16-year-old teenager living in London, Ontario, Canada, was forced to wait desperately for life-saving surgery. Julia suffers from a condition called valvular aortic stenosis – a narrow heart artery. Although Julia was born with the condition, when it was discovered, doctors informed her that an operation to relieve the artery should take place within five to eight weeks.[117] But it was not to be: her surgery was cancelled twice over a span of two months.

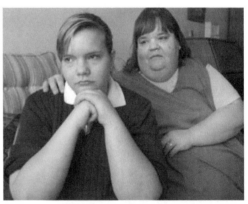

Credit: Sun Media Corp.

In February 2007, Julia's scheduled surgery at the Hospital for Sick Children in Toronto was cancelled the day before it was to be performed because the hospital lacked enough intensive care beds. "It is very, very stressful. They are messing with my daughter's life," said Colleen de Zeeuw, Julia's mother.[118]

Julia de Zeeuw (l), shown here with her mother Colleen, needed surgery to correct a dangerously narrowed heart artery, but it was repeatedly cancelled.

Coupled with the surgery's cancellation, having to travel to Toronto was a double frustration. The family had moved from the town of Arthur to London to be closer to the hospital where Julia's surgery was originally arranged to take place. However, soon after it relocated, the family was informed that all children's heart surgeries had been transferred to Toronto – approximately a two-hour drive from London. The family had not been told. "We would have never moved to London if we had known that," said Lloyd de Zeeuw, Julia's father.[119]

"Every child that is in our critical care unit requires a ventilator to breathe and specialty care. Sometimes when that happens… it means we have to reschedule other surgeries," explained Lisa Lipkin, hospital spokesperson at Sick Children.[120]

But for the de Zeeuws, the hospital's explanation was no comfort. Julia's surgery was rescheduled for April 24, but Sick Children cancelled it again. According to Colleen de Zeeuw, the hospital told the family that further tests showed she did not need immediate surgery. "This is not fair to my family. You can't mess with people's lives like that," said Colleen de Zeeuw.[121]

Meanwhile, the family was left hoping the hospital will eventually operate on Julia. "She will still need an operation, but we don't know when. It could be this year, next year or in five years," continued Colleen de Zeeuw. "We just have to live day to day and we will have to go through this all again."[122]

IN THE NICK OF TIME, CANADIAN CANCER SUFFERER TURNS TO U.S. DOCTORS

Once Sylvia de Vries realized that by the time she received anti-cancer treatment in Canada, if she received it at all, it might be too late, she and her husband, Adriaan, turned to the United States.

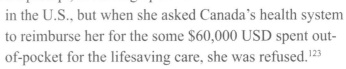

Thankfully, de Vries received a prompt, lifesaving operation – in the nick of time – in the U.S., but when she asked Canada's health system to reimburse her for the some $60,000 USD spent out-of-pocket for the lifesaving care, she was refused.[123]

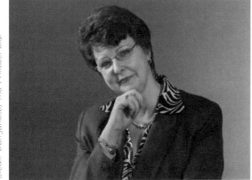

In 2004, de Vries was diagnosed with irritable bowel syndrome. Nevertheless, after two years, she sensed she had been misdiagnosed because she mysteriously gained weight. Seeking an alternative explanation, de Vries traveled to Detroit, Michigan's state-of-the-art Henry Ford Hospital for a CT scan.

Refusing to accept what effectively was a death-sentence-by-waiting-list in Canada, Sylvia de Vries traveled to Michigan for chemotherapy.

"We walked into emergency (in Detroit), and there was no wait, it was incredible," de Vries recalled.

Credit: Dan Janisse/The Windsor Star

The scan revealed that de Vries had ovarian cancer. "I was quite taken aback when they told me it was cancer," she said.

The test results should have alerted Canadian doctors that de Vries was in need of urgent treatment. Instead, de Vries would be shuffled around from doctor to doctor in Canada's publicly-provided health care system.

First, after she saw her family doctor – himself frustrated he could not speed along de Vries' treatment – de Vries learned she would need to have a CT scan done, but in Canada. This required her to see yet another doctor, a specialist, who referred her to a general surgeon, who, in turn, sent de Vries to a gynecologist. Then the gynecologist refused to see de Vries due to a perceived conflict of interest involving a colleague who previously had treated her.

"Less than an hour before my appointment I got a call from his office staff saying they would not see me," said de Vries. "[T]hat doctor sent a note… saying that I needed to see somebody in London [Ontario]."

The runaround was perplexing, but de Vries sensed she needed to be treated right away. Yet, there would be another immediate roadblock to overcome. The gynecologist – now the fourth Canadian doctor she had seen – told her he believed she did not have cancer.

"I was referred to a gynecologist out in the county and I saw him on the 16th of October [2006]," said de Vries. "He did an internal examination and sat down with my husband and I and said to the two of us, 'I do not believe that you have ovarian cancer.'"

Worried that she might soon die if she stayed in Canada, de Vries went back to Michigan. There Dr. Michael Hicks at St. Joseph Mercy Oakland hospital examined her on October 19. One week after the Canadian gynecologist assured de Vries she did not have cancer, Dr. Hicks removed a massive 18 kilograms of cancerous tissue and 13 liters of fluid. The operation claimed de Vries' ovaries, uterus, cervix, fallopian tubes and appendix.

According to Dr. Hicks, de Vries would have been in great danger if she waited even two more weeks for surgery. She faced "impending respiratory compromise with potential multi system failure requiring intensive medical support, thus rendering her unstable for surgery."

De Vries stayed in the U.S. for six courses of chemotherapy because there was a six-week wait at the local cancer center back in Windsor. The treatment in the U.S. cured her of the cancer, but it left de Vries and her husband with a staggering medical bill of $60,000. The financial strain was immense because treatment had to be paid up front.

"How did we pay for it? We drained all of our savings. We maxed out all of our credit cards," de Vries said.

The de Vrieses also had to open a line of credit to pay for the care. A spaghetti dinner fundraiser a friend hosted also raised $11,125 CAD (~$10,300 USD).[124]

With the cancer battle behind them, the de Vrieses turned to putting their financial house back in order. Unfortunately, this meant appealing to the government-run Ontario Health Insurance Plan, which refused to reimburse the $60,000 worth of out-of-country care because de Vries did not receive prior approval for financing.

"There's no question that Ms. De Vries required the medical service or she was going to die," argued Kate Sellar, de Vries' lawyer.[125] "She's being denied [a claim for reimbursement] basically because she didn't hand in the forms before she went for this urgent surgery," she also said.

SKIER WITH SEVERELY FRACTURED SHOULDER TOLD TO WAIT FOUR DAYS

Canadian Linda McDonough endured four days of agony waiting for surgery in a Canadian hospital after she badly damaged her shoulder in a skiing accident.

In February 2008, McDonough shattered her right humerus bone while skiing on vacation with her husband, Bill,[126] at Holiday Valley in Ellicottville, NY. The doctor at a local clinic, who X-rayed McDonough, recommended she have the fractured shoulder completely reconstructed.[127] Although immediate treatment there in the U.S. would relieve her pain, the McDonoughs decided against paying out-of-pocket for what would be major surgery. Instead, they drove back to Ontario to rely on their own government's universal health care system.

McDonough checked in to St. Catherines General Hospital, expecting emergency surgery to be performed relatively quickly, but, unknown to the McDonoughs, the government managed Niagara Health System in Ontario recently had implemented a four-category priority system for emergency surgeries.[128]

According to Canada's St. Catherines Standard, under the NHS's priority system, patients requiring emergency surgery are categorized as either A, B, C or D. The categories rank the perceived severity of a patient's condition. Wait times range from no wait to two hours for "Priority A" patients and two to seven days for those designated as "D" patients at the scale's other end.[129]

Morphine dulled McDonough's pain, but she had to endure not being able to eat or drink each day between 8 am and 4 pm in preparation for possible surgery. Coupled with an uncertain wait, the added discomfort of being without food or water "makes it doubly tough," said Bill McDonough.[130]

Finally, four days after the accident, McDonough's status was upgraded to "Priority B," which meant surgery should take place within two to eight hours.[131] That night, surgeons at last repaired – but did not reconstruct – McDonough's badly broken shoulder,[132] which was broken in three or four pieces.[133]

"I think it's unreasonable," declared Bill McDonough. "I always thought that in an emergency situation the system wasn't that bad, that you would be taken care of very quickly."[134]

The McDonoughs received little compassion for enduring such a lengthy wait. "It really is tough to wait, but there certainly are a number of procedures that can wait between two and seven days," said Patty Welychka, who directs the Niagara Health System's surgical program.[135]

DELAYED SURGICAL OP PATIENT FLIES TO INDIA FOR IMMEDIATE CARE

Flying to a faraway country for medical care did not seem too outrageous an idea for Canadian Raghav Shetty – at least, in comparison to the alternative. The 61-year-old Calgary, Alberta man's bum hip had effectively immobilized him. Yet he faced several years of waiting in distress for surgery in Canada's "universal" Medicare health system.[136]

Shetty had developed severe osteoarthritis in his left hip joint.[137] He was in so much pain that, even with the aid of painkillers, each step was tormenting.[138]

"I'm in extreme pain," he admitted. "I'm stuck at home, I can't work. It is difficult for me to provide financial support to my family and the quality of my life is very bad."[139]

"He can barely walk. He drags his legs everywhere he goes," added daughter, Shilpa Shetty.[140]

Shetty, a 20-year resident of Calgary, discovered the wait for partial hip replacement surgery would be up to two years. At the time, in 2004, some 25,000 patients were on waiting lists for surgery or diagnostic scans in Calgary's hospitals.[141]

Facing a bedridden wait on Medicare, Shetty and his wife, Prema, looked elsewhere for quicker treatment.[142] They discovered a private facility in Chennai, India offering immediate care.[143] The entire out-of-pocket cost for the operation and for both to fly to India would be $15,000 (CAD), but the couple believed waiting up to two years for care locally was not a realistic option.[144]

"I had no choice but to try elsewhere for my surgery due to the long waiting period and severe pain in my hip joint," Shetty said. "I could not walk more than a few meters. Under these conditions, waiting for one to two years was simply not possible for me."[145]

In September 2004, the Shettys traveled to Apollo Specialty Hospital for a successful five-hour surgery.[146] Shetty, an Indian immigrant, said returning to his native country for a medical procedure was not something he would have considered had it not been for the excessive wait.

"Of course, my first choice would have been always Canada," he said.[147] "However, in recent years, the waiting period for major surgeries is too long for patients suffering from severe pain and serious medical conditions."[148]

Daughter Shilpa objected to the tedious wait her father would have endured if he stayed in Canada. "We've given up on our health care system. Why don't they understand that some people are in so much pain that they just can't wait?" she asked. "We don't have any options and can't wait anymore."[149]

Though the long wait forced Shetty to look outside Canada, the health department in the province of Alberta rejected his claim for reimbursement for his care in India. Generally, the government reimburses only such patients who go abroad when treatment is unavailable locally or if the patient's life would be in jeopardy while waiting.[150]

As published in a 2007 Fraser Institute survey, an estimated 5,029 people in Alberta were waiting for hip or knee replacement surgery as of March 31, 2007.[151] According to the same report, nationwide some "estimated 523,600 Canadians had difficulties getting to see a specialist, 200,000 had difficulties getting non-emergency surgeries, and 294,800 had difficulties getting selected diagnostic tests."[152]

CANCER PATIENT TAKES ON CANADIAN HEALTH CARE BUREAUCRACY IN DESPERATE FIGHT TO LIVE

Suzanne Aucoin of St. Catharines, Ontario never imagined that dealing with the Canadian health care bureaucracy would be as tough as battling terminal cancer.

Aucoin had to go to the U.S. for treatment initially denied to her. While ill, she then engaged in a prolonged and complicated fight to get access to a life-extending anti-cancer drug and to recover the exorbitant amount she was forced to spend out of her own pocket on treatment.

In 1999, Aucoin was diagnosed with colorectal cancer. Surgeons removed large portions of her intestine and colon. But about four and a half years later, Aucoin became easily fatigued and felt pain in her side. A follow-up visit with her doctors revealed that the cancer had reappeared and spread to her lungs and liver.[153]

In January 2004, Aucoin began chemotherapy treatment for stage IV colon cancer, the most advanced stage. A CT scan showed that chemotherapy had been ineffective at destroying the tumor in her liver.[154] Aucoin's oncologist recommended that weekly doses of the powerful anti-cancer drug, Erbitux, offered her the best hope for staying alive. The problem was the drug – which can shrink tumors in advanced cancer patients – was not publicly-provided or even available for purchase in Ontario.[155]

Worse yet, Ministry of Health officials denied Aucoin's application for out-of-country funding to permit Aucoin to get the potentially life-extending drug in the U.S.[156] However, Aucoin claimed, the government was paying for three other patients with a similar form of cancer to receive treatment abroad. Reviews are on a case-by-case basis,[157] but the health ministry did confirm it paid for some patients to receive Erbitux in the U.S.[158]

"I just find it ridiculous that I have to go to these lengths when the government is glaringly wrong. They have all these inconsistencies, and I'm the one who suffers because of it," Aucoin said.[159]

Despite the government's refusal to fund her treatment, Aucoin began receiving weekly treatments of Erbitux at a cost of $14,000 (USD) a month at a clinic in West Seneca, NY.[160] The U.S. Food and Drug Administration approved Erbitux in February 2004.[161] Thankfully, friends and supporters raised more than $180,000 (CAD) over several years to help pay for her treatment.[162]

"You can't wait with this cancer," she said. "You can't wait for people to make decisions about your health. You can't wait for forms to be filled out. You have to go where the drug is."[163]

In fall 2005, Health Canada – the Canadian agency responsible for evaluating drugs – approved Erbitux.[164] But health officials refused to cover Erbitux and limited the number of patients who could have access.[165]

Fortunately, a loophole existed. In December 2005, Aucoin was the first patient allowed Erbitux under a Special Access Program set up for seriously ill patients. She would have to pay over $6,000 (CAD) a month for treatment, which she received at a Hamilton, Ontario clinic,[166] while the government paid the administrative costs.[167]

"I just want to take care of myself," Aucoin said. "My job is to get well and I feel like my government's letting me down because they're not doing their job."[168]

Following another appeal for out-of-country funding several months later, the government changed its mind and, without explanation, agreed to cover Aucoin's treatment.[169] The decision meant Aucoin would no longer pay out-of-pocket, but she would again need to travel across the border. Oddly, the government directed her to a Buffalo, NY cancer hospital that charged thousands of dollars more for Erbitux than the West Seneca clinic Aucoin used for out-of-pocket treatment.[170] She began treatment at the Roswell Park Cancer Institute in April 2006.[171]

Then the Ontario government stonewalled Aucoin's attempt to be reimbursed. In June 2006, health officials denied her application for reimbursement saying the government would "only approve [reimbursement] if it's in a certain setting, i.e., a hospital," not a private clinic. Moreover, Aucoin was not granted funding approval before she went abroad for treatment.[172]

"I am completely disgusted with our health care system," Aucoin said. "I am very discouraged and frustrated by the lack of professionalism, the lack of consistency and the lack of care for me as an individual patient."[173] She added, "I'm not asking for Botox, I'm asking for life-saving treatment."[174]

After losing on appeal and running out of options,[175] Aucoin appealed to Ontario's ombudsman, Andre Martin. Following his investigation, in January 2007 Ontario's health officials finally agreed to pay over $76,000 (CAD) for Aucoin's out-of-country care and for legal expenses.[176] The ombudsman blasted health officials for their "cruel" treatment and "slavish adherence to rules at the expense of common sense."[177]

"I should never have had to deal with this, it takes all my energy to fight cancer," Aucoin said. "It rights a wrong on some levels but you cannot put a price tag on my mental strain and stress."[178]

Tragically, Aucoin lost her fight against cancer. She passed away in November 2007.[179]

IMMIGRANT RETURNS TO NATIVE COUNTRY FOR CANCER TREATMENT

A 14-week wait for cancer surgery prompted Branislav Djukic, an immigrant hailing from the former Yugoslavia, to fly back to his native country to pay for private care.[180]

The London, Ontario man first went to the emergency room in November 2003, complaining of back pain. Though an ultrasound showed no sign of an abnormality, he returned to the hospital an additional two times over the next two months in pain. Djukic's doctors suspected he was suffering from back spasms and a urinary tract infection.

In April 2004, Djukic discovered blood in his urine. He was referred to a urology clinic in London where, in June, an ultrasound revealed a lesion thought to be cancerous. A follow-up CT scan in late September showed he had renal cell cancer. Though doctors established the cause of the ailment, Djukic faced waiting until January 2005 – 14 weeks and three days away – for an operation.

"I felt very bad," Djukic said. "I couldn't believe that in a rich country, you had to wait so long."

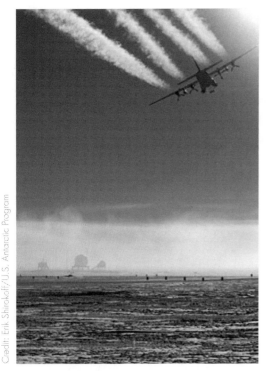

Credit: Erik Shirokoff/U.S. Antarctic Program

A 14-week wait for cancer surgery in Canada prompted Branislav Djukic, an immigrant from the former Yugoslavia, to fly to Belgrade for private care.

Djukic appealed to the Ontario government, which was his provincial health care provider, to pay him to get the care he needed right away by going abroad for surgery. However, the health bureaucrats refused this request in January 2005, determining that Djukic's prognosis was unlikely to change during the wait.

"We were very confused, we didn't know what to do," Djukic said. "I was lost."

Instead of taking a risk, Djukic flew to Belgrade – from which he had fled in 1995 – to have part of his left kidney removed. He paid $5,000 (CAD) out-of-pocket for the surgery and another $5,000 (CAD) for travel and accommodation.

"Canada prides itself in being one of the best countries in the world to live in and this is one of the reasons we came here," said daughter Maja Djukic. "However, in a time of need for somebody in my dad's situation, Yugoslavia offered better and faster treatment. They could not understand that they would make you wait that long to treat a disease of such seriousness in a country such as Canada and neither could we."

Maja Djukic initiated an appeal for her father to receive compensation for his medical costs abroad. In January 2007, it was reported that the Ontario Health Services Appeal and Review Board sided with Djukic, ruling, "a delay in obtaining treatment… would result in medically significant, irreversible tissue damage." The Board ordered the Ontario government to reimburse Djukic for the cost of surgery – but not for his other expenses.

HOOKED ON PRESCRIPTION MEDICATION WHILE WAITING FOR SURGERY

Canadian Susan Warner became addicted to doctor-prescribed painkillers while enduring 16 months waiting for knee replacement surgery.

Warner, a self-employed photographer from Calgary, blew out her knee in

September 2003. The injury was so severe that there was not any cartridge left. An X-ray revealed that Warner needed to have her knee replaced, but the surgeon she was referred to said it would take 12 to 18 months to receive a new knee.[181]

"At that point, I just couldn't believe it because it was excruciatingly painful," Warner said.[182] "It's inhuman. The quality of my life is horrible and there's absolutely nothing I can do about it."[183]

To cope with the pain, Warner began taking medication while waiting for her number to be called at Rockyview General Hospital.[184] She started on Tylenol 3s – Codeine – then moved to Percocet. Despite the risk of dependency, Warner had little choice but to take the doctor-prescribed medication to continue making a living.[185]

"I couldn't take the luxury of not working," Warner, who is single, explained. "If I would have stopped working, I would have lost everything I own."[186]

After a few weeks taking Percocet, Warner strongly suspected she was developing a dependency.[187] "When I wake up in the morning, I'm shaking and have headaches," she said.[188]

With little prospect of a timely surgery in Canada and dealing with the twin burden of a busted knee and an addiction, Warner looked elsewhere for treatment. Unfortunately, no private clinic in Canada she approached agreed to operate on her. The $25,000 (USD) price tag for care in the U.S. was more than Warner could afford.[189]

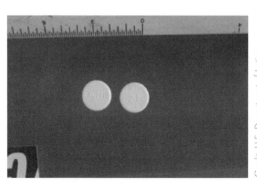

Credit: U.S. Department of Justice

Canadian Susan Warner became addicted to doctor-prescribed painkillers while waiting 16 months for knee replacement surgery.

"After a few months of this [waiting in pain], I would have done anything I could," Warner confessed. "It wasn't easy living, taking a drug every morning, waking up and taking a drug to feel normal."[190]

Warner described living with the addiction as "absolute hell." Her bones would ache and legs spasm. She found it difficult to get sleep and keep warm. "The drug ha[d] just completely taken over the body," she said.[191]

Finally, she received knee surgery in January 2005.[192] But her ordeal was not over. After receiving a new knee, she was told she would have to wait another six months for detoxification treatment.[193]

Warner contrasted her experience in Canada's government-managed health care system to finding relatively easy access to care during her time living in the U.S. and Germany. "Both times [there] I've had absolutely no problem getting health care," she said.[194]

However, the wait in Canada took a tremendous toll on all aspects of her life. "I paid dearly… my health, my finances, everything was put on hold for two, almost three years," she said.[195]

"It's left my life shallow, and I'm angry, and it's going to take a bit of time for me to rebuild," she added. "I just hope I'm never injured again or need to use their [Canadian Medicare's] resources in this way."[196]

YOU CAN'T EAT, YOU CAN'T TALK, YOU CAN'T MOVE YOUR JAW AT ALL – BUT YOU MUST WAIT THREE MONTHS FOR TREATMENT

One day, while eating a chicken leg, Canadian Diane Nesenbrink, then 13, encountered what would become a life-long affliction. She heard a crack and her jaw locked into place while still open. In pain, Nesenbrink tried forcing her mouth shut, but that proved extremely difficult.[197]

"I looked like a Pac-Man with his mouth open ready to gobble things up… except I couldn't move my mouth," Nesenbrink said in 2007, looking back on the experience 27 years ago.

Despite the continuous problem restricting her jaw movement, Nesenbrink's doctor was unhelpful.

"My doctor told me it was all in my head," Nesenbrink recalled. "But I couldn't chew, I couldn't smile and I was in pain."

Finally, Nesenbrink went to her dentist, who diagnosed her with temporomandibular joint syndrome (TMJ). According to Canada's Globe and Mail, the condition affects one out of every seven people. For most people, it causes temporary, minor issues. However, in one percent of cases, TMJ requires jaw joint replacement surgery.

"We see patients who are in dire straits: Talking, eating, chewing, smiling are all difficult, if not impossible," Dr. Gerald Baker of Mount Sinai Hospital in Toronto told the Globe and Mail. "The condition can be debilitating."

However, for those suffering from severe TMJ, the wait time in Canada for a joint replacement is just as frustrating as living with the condition. In fact, the average wait can be over two years. Those in critical need of surgery because they cannot move their mouths must wait a minimum of three months.

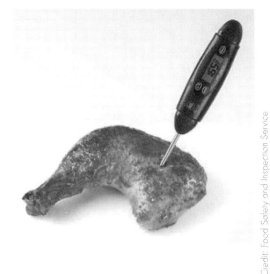

Strangely, joint replacement operations on other parts of the body, such as a hip or knee, are guaranteed to be complete within nine months, including the consultation and subsequent surgery.

Diane Nesenbrink's jaw locked open after she bit into a chicken leg, but her doctor told her she was imagining it.

"It's the same idea as a hip or a knee – the joint gets damaged and needs to be replaced," said Dr. Baker. "The jaw joint is an important joint as well, but we've been forgotten... Doing [joint replacement] sooner is a good investment and it helps patients avoid the vicious cycle of chronic pain."

As for Nesenbrink, she underwent numerous operations, which included replacing her jaw joint with cartilage and rib bone. In 1999, finally, she received a plastic and metal replacement for her jaw. Because the prosthetic lasts only seven to 10 years, Nesenbrink had a replacement done in October 2006.

Many other patients are forced to wait. In 2007, there were some 50 people in Ontario waiting for TMJ replacement. There is intense competition for slots because Ontario has only one hospital, Mount Sinai, that offers full joint jaw replacement surgery, and it has a budget of only $210,000 (CAD) (~$193,600 USD) annually to commit to all such operations.

BRAIN CANCER PATIENT DENIED LAST-CHANCE DRUG DESPITE SPECIALISTS' RECOMMENDATIONS

Cancer patient Chad Curley was given hope when he learned that a blend of brain tumor-fighting drugs could possibly extend his life. The problem: the government in Canada's government health care system refused to pay for the drugs that offered Chad his last and best opportunity to survive.

Ironically, the drug Chad needed was, in fact, government-approved in Canada[198] – but not covered for fighting the particular form of cancer afflicting Chad.[199]

Chad's long battle against a stage two-to-three brain tumor began when he was diagnosed in June 2003.[200] The bout with cancer forced the 37-year-old autoworker from Windsor, Ontario to quit his job at the Chrysler Canada assembly plant. It would paralyze his left side and confine him to a wheelchair.[201]

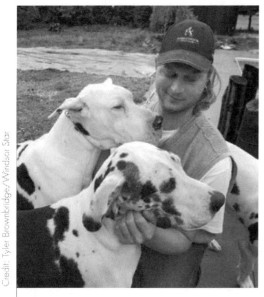

In June 2003, Chad underwent a craniotomy operation. One year later, the operation was repeated. He also underwent several years of radiation and traditional chemotherapy treatment. But in the fall of 2007, a MRI scan showed an increase of tumor activity and suggested that the tumor had become resistant to chemotherapy drugs.[202]

Additional surgery was impractical, so Chad and his wife, Meira, looked for alternative treatments. Through their own Internet research, the couple learned of a powerful treatment that involved a two-drug cocktail of Avastin and CPT11. The treatment had been shown to reduce the size of brain tumors.[203]

The Canadian health system refused to approve Chad Curley for Avastin to fight his brain cancer.

Chad obtained three written opinions from specialists in London (Ontario), Detroit and Cleveland recommending the cocktail treatment. The problem Chad faced was that the government health care system in Ontario refused to fund Chad's treatment.[204] The government had Avastin on its approved-drugs list – but not for combating brain cancer.[205]

The financial burden for the Curleys to buy Avastin themselves would be tremendous. The drug carries a price tag of $5,000 (CAD) (~$4,600 USD) for each treatment. Chad faced the need for three courses initially to determine its effectiveness;[206] thereafter, he would need to continue the treatment every two weeks.[207]

Chrysler refused to release Chad's pension,[208] and Chad's supplemental insurance would not pay for the drugs he desperately needed.[209]

"We get shoved away from everywhere we go," Meira Curley said. "I've already taken out a second mortgage. I'm just not going to let something happen to him without a fight."[210]

The couple and their friends managed to raise enough money to fund the first course of treatment, which occurred in mid-November 2007[211] at the Windsor Regional Cancer Centre.[212] The second round, again at Windsor Regional, in late November had to be charged to a credit card.[213]

"It has to be paid by January but I'll worry about it then," Meira said at the time.[214]

According to Meira, the results were promising. "You can see he has more feeling on the left [paralyzed] side," she said soon after Chad's second treatment. "You can see he's starting to improve."[215]

The government health system still refused to provide Avastin for Chad, despite Meira's appeal to Ontario's then Minister of Health, George Smitherman MPP.[216] A fundraiser was held to help with the escalating medical bills,[217] but, regrettably, Chad passed away on February 21, 2008.[218]

Meira wrote on a website dedicated to her husband's struggle: "He touched many people throughout his life and will always be remembered with love... Rest well my Sweetie."

CANADIAN DOCTORS HOLD LOTTERIES - "WINNING" PATIENTS LOSE THEIR DOCTORS

Winning the lottery is usually a cause for celebration. However, for some long-standing Canadian patients awaiting treatment on the government's health care wait list, 'winning' the health care lottery can result not in treatment but in being dropped entirely from a doctor's practice.

In Canada, demand for government-managed health services is high, but the supply of doctors is dwindling.[219] In fact, more than some four million Canadians do not have a primary doctor, forcing many in need of medical attention to seek out alternative treatment centers or emergency room care.[220]

Still, thousands of patients are stuck on waiting lists for necessary treatment.[221] As a result, some Canadian doctors faced with large patient loads have turned to lotteries in order to select at random patients to drop from their practice.[222]

Janet Gauthier, 53, is one such patient bumped off her doctor's roster. In July 2008, she received a notice by mail that Dr. Ken Runciman had cut her from his practice in Powassan, Ontario.[223]

"He could have done it a different way," Gauthier said.[224]

Dr. Runciman explained that his rationale for eliminating roughly 100 patients in two drawings was an objective way to thin an overstretched practice.[225]

"It was just my way of trying to minimize the bias… rather than going through the list and saying 'I don't like you, and I don't like you,'" he said. "There is only a certain number of people I can see in a day. My day is already 11 hours and I don't care for it being longer."[226]

Runciman is not the only Canadian doctor using a lottery to drop patients. Canada's National Post has reported several such instances:

> A new family practice in Newfoundland held a lottery last month [July 2008] to pick its caseload from among thousands of applicants. An Edmonton doctor selected names randomly earlier this year to pare 500 people from his heavy caseload. And in Ontario, regulators have heard reports of a number of other physicians also using draws to choose, or remove, patients.[227]

Moreover, according to Gauthier, in some cases the lottery system removes elderly patients. "Everybody was kind of mad about it," she said.[228] "Everybody thinks it's a joke."[229]

As for Gauthier, she was able to register with a different doctor in Callander, but she was not pleased about driving 11 miles further during bad winter weather to see her new doctor.[230]

IN CANADA, PROTESTING WAITING LISTS CAN GET YOU BUMPED FROM SURGERY

Carly Lamont of British Columbia, Canada is a 12-year-old disabled teenager on an 18-month waiting list for spinal surgery. She suffers from severe scoliosis (curvature of the spine), a condition that could adversely affect her internal organs if not addressed. For months, her family protested the surgery delay to help Carly get the care she needed.[231]

Instead, after drawing public attention to Carly's situation, the province's only two orthopedic surgeons capable of operating on a child terminated their treatment for Carly.[232]

Carly suffers not only from severe scoliosis but also epilepsy and cerebral palsy.[233] As of February 2009, her spine was curved at 90 degrees.,[234] The condition is so severe that Carly's organs are in danger of being crushed, and she is 40 degrees over a typical surgery candidate. To keep her spine in place, Carly has worn a back brace since age seven.[235]

"At seven years of age, our daughter had to begin wearing a back brace 22 hours a day to help her spine from worsening and has worn these and also two stints in back casts done under General Anesthetic 24 hours a day for six weeks at a time right up until March of this year [2008]," elaborated Susan Watson, Carly's mother.[236]

In February 2008, Carly was added to the 18-month waiting list for surgery. According to Watson, Dr. Firoz Miyanji, the orthopedic specialist, said that despite his recommendation that Carly should soon have surgery she "would be at the end of an 18 month waitlist for surgery as you don't put Peter in front of Paul." Carly "could wait like everyone else," Watson further wrote.[237]

The delay was frightening for the family. "We have been told by Carly's orthopedic surgeon that her spine will deteriorate during this time," wrote Watson in the Vancouver Sun. "She is at 70 degrees now. At 90 degrees organs can begin to be damaged" by the spine crushing them.[238]

Alarmed, Watson initiated a campaign to draw attention to her daughter's plight. She wrote letters about the horrendous wait her daughter faced to top government officials, including Prime Minister Stephen Harper and British Columbia Premier Gordon Campbell, as well as health ministers and hospital administrators. She launched an Internet petition and wrote in the Vancouver Sun asking for assistance.[239]

However, Watson's public protests, instead of pressuring the hospital into action, received a hostile reaction.

"One of the doctors had gotten angry at me for doing so at a meeting we had at the beginning of May 2008," she wrote in the Internet petition. "I told them all (including Donna Gerelle – a higher up at the hospital) that in no way was I going to stop contacting the government or media and that it had nothing to do with them as people or their skills as surgeons…"[240]

In the summer of 2008, at a routine follow-up appointment for Carly, the family learned in writing that the hospital's orthopedic surgeons would no longer treat Carly except in a case of emergency. Instead, they would refer the family to a pediatric specialist in Edmonton or Calgary because of differences with Carly's parents.[241]

"I was shocked, absolutely stunned," said David Lamont, Carly's father.[242]

The letter, which was signed by Dr. Chris Reilly, Head of the Department of Pediatric Orthopedics at B.C. Children's Hospital, and Dr. Miyanji, read in part:

> There have been many communications regarding Carly's care both through our offices, the hospital administration and also public media, including newspapers and the recent website… We feel that we have not been able to establish a therapeutic relationship with your family that will allow us to care for Carly.[243]

The two doctors are the only specialists in British Columbia that perform spinal surgery on a child.[244] As a result, the family is faced with traveling outside British Columbia to get Carly surgery – something they wish could be avoided.

"We do not want to travel out of B.C. to have this done," Watson wrote. "We are residents of British Columbia and pay our taxes. It is an extremely delicate and dangerous surgery, especially for kids with Cerebral Palsy…"

Watson also wrote that post-op treatment will require "a year's worth of recovery" and many follow-up examinations. "This would mean us traveling back and forth between wherever we could find a new specialist outside of B.C. to help Carly and then who knows how long of a waitlist she will be put on then?" wrote Watson.[245]

Carly is one of 150 children in British Columbia waiting for spinal surgery.[246] During a seven-week stretch in the spring of 2008, the B.C. Children's Hospital cancelled at least 25 surgeries because of a shortage of intensive care nurses.[247]

Meanwhile, the family is trying to mend differences at the hospital.[248]

CANADIAN SHUNNED AT HOME OPTS FOR SURGERY ABROAD

Jill Misangyi spent 16 years waiting in Canada for surgery to relieve chronic back pain.[249] The 49-year-old nurse from Hamilton, Ontario desperately needed spinal surgery but could not get approved for surgery. Then, when she developed a dependency on painkilling medication while waiting, Canadian doctors refused to operate on her.

Out of options in Canada and her back getting worse, Misangyi found a way to bypass government-managed Canadian Medicare by flying to India for top-notch, affordable care right away.

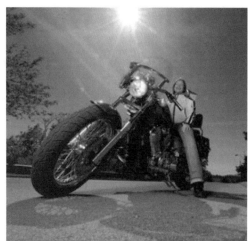

After being involved in three car accidents in one year while in her 30s, Misangyi was nearly crippled. The daily pain she experienced was so intense that getting out of bed was difficult. Misangyi needed a spinal fusion and laminectomy performed, but the years of enduring chronic backache combined with a heavy dosage of painkillers and physiotherapy had worn her down.

But Canadian doctors refused to agree that her condition warranted surgery. "I had many MRIs over the past two years and they always said it wasn't bad enough to operate on," Misangyi said in 2007.

After waiting 16 years for surgery in Canada to relieve chronic back pain, Jill Misangyi flew to India for private treatment.

To make matters worse, Misangyi then realized she had become addicted to the prescribed painkillers. As a result, Canadian doctors refused to operate, telling Misangyi that she was not eligible for a surgery that had only a 20 percent chance of improving her condition.

"It got to the point where it was so bad that my pain medication had increased so much that it was affecting my work life," Misangyi said. She recalled that even the private doctors in Canada she contacted "thought I was drug-dependent and too high a risk for them."[250]

"There are a lot of people in Canada suffering with back pain and it's very hard to get surgery there," Misangyi said. "Waiting lists just to see specialists are 6 months to a couple of years, and another couple of years before or if they will do the surgery on you."[251]

But Misangyi discovered how to get the care she needed immediately – and at a fraction of what it would have cost in a U.S. hospital. To her delight, the Wockhardt Hospital in Bangalore, India agreed to the surgery in July 2007 for less than $12,000.

That figure included airfare for her and a companion, as well as hospital and hotel accommodation and expenses.[252] Moreover, the hospital issued a partial refund when the actual cost of the operation was less than charged.

Misangyi never believed she would be flying around the world as a medical tourist. But she raved about her experience.

"It was a wonderful experience. I've got my life back. The medical team – the doctors, the nurses and everybody right down to the housekeeping staff, is just wonderful. They make you feel very warm," she said. "I would most definitely recommend it [medical tourism] highly to anybody."

Moreover, by going abroad, Misangyi added, "I'm saving the Canadian medical system money."

Misangyi was back at work as a nurse five weeks after surgery. The decision to get care in India rejuvenated her life, and Misangyi is able to celebrate that on a new motorcycle she bought that not long ago would be unthinkable for her to be on.

"I have been off all pain medication for at least 9 months and am back exercising building muscle," she said. "I really do have a second chance at life."

PAINTER'S AILING HANDS NOT REASON ENOUGH FOR SPEEDY SURGERY

Australian Peter Horne wanted nothing more than to get on with his career as a professional painter, but the 61-year-old's wish was put on hold because rheumatoid arthritis disabled his hands, as well as his shoulder and left ankle.[1]

Horne waited painfully for reconstructive surgery to rebuild his hands so he could get back to his beloved profession, but on two occasions, the Royal Melbourne Hospital in Parkville, Australia, an inner-city suburb in northern Melbourne, cancelled scheduled treatment. In April 2007, after Horne had been waiting two years, the hospital let a tentative appointment pass without notifying Horne.

"You get your hopes up and they [the public health administrators] say: 'We will put you on for so and so,' but we have been shunted off," says Horne.

According to the Australian government's health care guidelines, surgeons should have treated Horne relatively quickly. As a "category two" patient, the second-most severe designation, Horne's condition qualified him for "[a]dmission within 90 days… for a condition causing some pain, dysfunction or disability but which is not likely to deteriorate quickly, or become an emergency."[2]

The sad reality is that Horne could expect to wait indefinitely. Under Australia's rationing of public health services, Horne's ailment is not judged severe enough to warrant a speedy operation.

"Our priorities need to be trauma cases and the urgent cases," explained Dr. Christine Kilpatrick, executive director of the Royal Melbourne's clinical governance department. "There are some patients who do unfortunately wait for long periods of time: clearly they are not the most urgent cases."

Today, Horne has difficulty not only handling a paintbrush, but also performing daily tasks like dressing himself. His deteriorating condition forced him to quit his job teaching art at the Alamein Community Centre. Horne attempted to practice his craft by holding a paintbrush using both hands – an inadequate, temporary solution at best. "I just want to be able to get out there and contribute: I want to work for another 15 years," he said.

82-HOUR AGONY FOR ELDERLY HOSPITAL PATIENT

Rita Robins, an 81-year-old widow and retiree, suffered 82 hours in pain at a Western Australia public hospital after a fall fractured her left hip.[3]

On the night she fell, Robins' family took her to Royal Perth Hospital, but instead of receiving urgent medical attention, the elderly great-grandmother would endure two cancelled surgeries and spend the next 82 hours waiting in agony, unable to move.

Upon arriving at the hospital at 11:45 pm on a Tuesday, Robins was placed on a gurney to prevent her from moving the injured hip. She was carted away to "empty spots" in the hospital and promised surgery the next morning, but, that Wednesday at 1:30 pm, Robins instead was taken to what a family member described as a "holding pen."

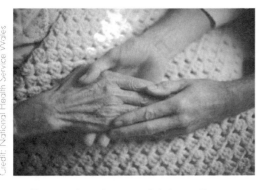

Staff at Royal Perth Hospital did not offer Rita Robins, 81, a helping hand when it forced her to wait 82 hours for treatment for a fractured hip (model shown).

"This was just stretchers again with curtains between them in just one big open room," recalled daughter-in-law Dianne Robins. "[B]ecause she's on her back, they had to put a catheter in for her because she can't get up to go to the toilet or anything."

An immobile Robins would remain on the gurney all day Wednesday.

Diane Robins requested food and medicine for her mother-in-law, but was told no one was available to help. She explained, "I requested that if the operation wasn't going to happen, could they feed her because she had been fasting from the night before, and could they give her some of the medication she usually takes... But the nurse just straight out said to me, 'I can't find anybody to come and do what we need to do.'"

At 2:30 pm on Thursday - approaching 39 hours since her arrival at the hospital - Robins was moved to a bed. Then Thursday's surgery was cancelled because of pre-existing conditions, according to a hospital spokeswoman. A worn-out Robins, who suffers from dementia, continued to be unable to eat or to sleep. "She was really tired, she didn't sleep all night, she was scared and with all this stress, it made her mind wander because she also hadn't eaten," explained Dianne Robins.

At last, on Friday at 9:30 am, surgeons operated to repair Robins' badly injured hip. "[F]rom the time she got to the hospital, until the operation, that's about 82 hours of her lying on her back, not being able to move," said Dianne Robins. "I don't think you would do this to an animal."

BOY SUFFERS HEARING LOSS BECAUSE OF EAR SURGERY DELAYS

An eight-year-old boy from Warnbro, Western Australia lost half of his hearing in one ear because he was forced to wait nearly a year for routine ear surgery.

Kyle Inglis was diagnosed in June 2006 with a tumor in his left ear. The boy suffers from cholesteatoma, a skin growth that can result in bone loss in the ear and lead to deafness and even brain infection.[4]

An operation that takes half an hour to complete was scheduled for November 2006, but was cancelled because a surgical microscope was unavailable.[5] Then, a second surgery, scheduled for April 2007, was cancelled because the special microscope was in use at a different hospital.[6]

At last, after a newspaper publicized the boy's situation, doctors operated in May 2007. However, Kyle's doctors at Fremantle Hospital discovered that the long wait had, unfortunately, allowed the cyst in the ear to become inflamed. This required the removal of destroyed ear bone.[7]

"[W]e've been told by doctors that the reason it got so serious is because it has taken so long to be done and I'm angry about this," said the boy's furious mother, Tracey Balkham. "How many other kids and adults are waiting?"[8]

Balkham maintains that the government-managed health system long has failed her son. Inglis' hearing has steadily deteriorated since 2002 but doctors erroneously believed he merely suffered from glue ear,[9] a painless condition in which fluid collects behind the eardrum. She adds that hearing loss stunted her son's verbal and educational development.[10]

"This has definitely held his education back and held back his speech at an important part of his development," she said. "He's got to sit up [at] the front in class, he's had ear infections in between, because of leakage from the cyst and we have to yell at him so he can hear us."[11]

Kyle had to be scheduled for reconstructive surgery to repair his ear.

"This poor boy is a victim of our health system in crisis," exclaimed parliamentarian Dr. Kim Hames, then Shadow Minister for Health.[12] "It's pretty bloody disgraceful that a poor little kid had to have a section of bone removed in his ear because he had to wait so long in our health system and now has to go back and get another operation to repair the defect."[13]

Kyle's dealing with the public health system is not an isolated case. According to the Australian Sunday Times, in 2007 there were roughly 1,000 children in Western Australia "waiting up to 642 days for ear, nose and throat operations."[14]

NO BEDS TO DELIVER STILLBORN BABY

Zareen Nisha of Merrylands, Australia faced what no mother ever should: the baby she was carrying died in her womb. To compound the bereaved woman's suffering, there was not an open bed available at a major Australian public hospital for her to deliver her stillborn son. Instead, Nisha was directed to go home with the full knowledge that her unborn child was no longer living.[15]

Nisha's appalling care began months before, in November 2006. After her general practitioner discovered she was pregnant, it took 12 weeks for Nisha to be seen for a prenatal appointment at Westmead Hospital's University Clinic. Although Nisha believed she was a high-risk pregnancy because of a history of reproductive complications, the health care system was breathtakingly inattentive to the 36-year-old's needs.

For instance, doctors administered only one ultrasound evaluation during her pregnancy - at 20 weeks - despite her age. Moreover, when Nisha became concerned her baby was at risk of having Down syndrome, no test was performed at the clinic. Eventually, she paid out of her own pocket for a private test.

Tragically, by the time doctors discovered the baby was in danger, it was too late to save him. In April 2007, at seven months pregnant, Nisha's doctor noticed a problem and sent her to Westmead. Despite the doctor notifying the hospital of her impending arrival and need for urgent attention, Nisha was told to wait nearly 30 minutes. At last, a test revealed that the umbilical cord had wrapped around the baby's neck twice and killed him.

"There was no disability or anything - he died because the cord had coiled around his neck," Nisha explained. "Ultrasounds would have picked up that he was becoming tangled in the cord... If they had seen it [the cord] was tangling they would have saved him - I believe if they had done more ultrasounds they would have seen that," she said.

Despite the tragic circumstance, hospital staff said that "there were no beds" available for Nisha to deliver her stillborn son. She would have to return when space became available. At 2 am the next day, Nisha went back to the hospital to give birth to her son, Aahil, around 8 pm.

Following her ordeal, Nisha had strong words to say about Australia's government-managed health care service. She compared it to that of her native Fiji, where she had delivered her first child nine years previously.

"The standard of care is higher in Fiji then it is here," she said emphatically.

PUBLIC HOSPITAL IGNORES WOMAN, WHO MISCARRIES IN HOSPITAL BATHROOM

At six weeks pregnant, 19-year-old Rachel Murray was taken to the hospital suffering bleeding and abdominal pain. After a lengthy wait for a doctor and eventual discharge, the Cranbourne, Australian woman had to be rushed back the same day when her condition deteriorated. Yet, instead of attending to her, hospital staff left Murray alone to have a miscarriage in the hospital's public bathroom.[16]

At about 11:30 am, fiancé Shane Simons took Murray to Casey Hospital, a public facility in Berwick, Australia. Murray was bleeding and in some discomfort, but she was left to wait for at least 90 minutes before a doctor examined her.[17]

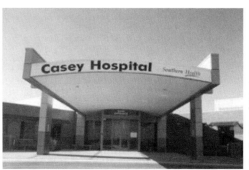

The doctor recommended that Murray have an ultrasound, but the hospital could not provide the exam for her at the time,[18] despite it having the equipment to perform such a screening.[19] Instead, the couple was told to go home and to return if Murray's pain continued.[20]

Unable to get medical attention from Casey Hospital in Berwick, Australia, Rachel Murray suffered a miscarriage in the hospital's public bathroom.

The bleeding and pain became more severe later that evening, and an ambulance was called to rush Murray back to the hospital at 7 pm.[21] However, yet again, instead of receiving urgent medical attention, Murray was left in the hospital's waiting area reportedly for up to two hours.[22] Humiliated, Murray said she felt hospital staff treated her like "spare change."[23]

"It was really upsetting. We felt like no one was looking after us. She was bleeding in the waiting room in front of everyone else," Simons said. "They could have given Rachel the dignity of a private room."[24]

Before a doctor attended to her, Murray went to the bathroom, where she had a spontaneous miscarriage. A doctor finally saw her around 8:15 pm.[25]

"When I saw the fetus I almost fainted," Murray recalled.[26]

Though Murray's ordeal was painful and humiliating, hospital administrators defended the treatment as "appropriate clinical care."[27] Siva Sivarajah, executive director of acute services for the public Southern Adelaide Health Service (Southern Health), reasoned in a subsequent assessment, "Unfortunately there is no clinical intervention to prevent an inevitable miscarriage in the very early stages of pregnancy... It is Southern Health's priority to provide women going through such an incident with high quality clinical care and support, which was provided in the case referred to."[28]

It is no surprise that Murray and Simmons feel let down by the government-managed health care system.

"I think it was disgusting the way they treated her," blasted Simons. "No woman should have to go through that."[29]

ELDERLY WOMAN WAITS NEARLY FOUR YEARS FOR CATARACT SURGERY

A wait of nearly four years for cataract surgery was a living hell for Nellie de Bomford. The smallest amount of light caused the 83-year-old retiree from Acton, Australia extreme discomfort. Yet, until her situation was exposed in the media, the government-managed health service would not fit her in for a 20-minute procedure that would improve her life immensely.[30]

In June 2004, de Bomford had cataract surgery on one of her eyes. She expected to have the cataract removed on her other eye within 12 months, but after she was put on the "elective surgery" waiting list, her referral to a specialist expired. De Bomford's appointment was then, essentially, forgotten about until late 2007, when a specialist estimated the procedure would not take place until sometime in 2009.

Meanwhile, the cataract was extremely disruptive. The blinds in de Bomford's home had to be closed because the glare would blind her. Makeshift cataract glasses made of sunglasses put overtop prescription lenses were of little use for getting around indoors. On more than one occasion, de Bomford fell, at one point, requiring 10 stitches to her forehead.

"At the moment her life is hell. When she gets to a door and the light hits her it's just bang and then she can't see," said daughter, Suzanne Cowell, who lives with de Bomford to care for her. "Our home is always dark and mum gets very frustrated. Life is pretty miserable for her," she added.

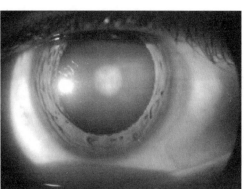

Nellie de Bomford, 83, waited almost four years for a 20-minute cataract operation (model shown).

What is frustrating, said Cowell, is her mother would be "as good as gold" if she had the simple procedure, but de Bomford is forced to wait for the government-managed health service to get around to helping her because she cannot afford the over $2,000 AUD (~$1,650 USD) price tag for a private operation.

"It's a terrible thing for me to say, but I did tell the clinic staff that if she's dead when they finally get around to getting the surgery done will they then dig her up for it," said Cowell. "My mother is 83 years old and I am disgusted how the aged are treated in this state."

Fortunately, after Cowell wrote to the local press about her mother's wait, less than a week later a public hospital, North West Regional, sprang into action.[31] The hospital's chief executive, Jane Holden, intervened to get de Bomford a scheduled cataract operation in early May 2008.[32]

"I feel on top of the world about it but I am still worried about the other people still waiting," de Bomford said.[33]

BUSY MIDWIVES ELSEWHERE AS HUSBAND CATCHES BABY BORN IN HOSPITAL BATHROOM

Kathy Patsidis, a 41-week-pregnant Meadowbank,[34] Australia woman, was left unattended to give birth with no anesthetic in a hospital bathroom. Despite her frantic pleas to midwives too busy to provide pain relief, Mrs. Patsidis was left alone with only her husband, Nick, by her side to catch their baby when she suddenly went into labor.

The ordeal began at 7 am in early May 2008, when Patsidis went to the maternity ward at Royal North Shore Hospital in Sydney. It took two-and-a half hours to admit Patsidis to a room,[35] though her contractions were 10 minutes apart.[36] After finally securing a room, the couple was effectively abandoned thereafter.

The couple complained that midwives offered little assistance; instead, they were told repeatedly that staff were "too busy" to monitor Patsidis.[37] They asked for an epidural 90 minutes before her water broke, but were told "the anesthetist is too busy" to administer one. They report that the anesthetist "never showed up."[38]

"She was in a state of rage… she told the midwife, not once but twice, it feels like… there's a bowling ball coming out of me," said Nick Patsidis.[39] He added, "The midwife's not done anything, just held my wife there, not done an internal examination or anything."[40]

Suddenly, his wife went into labor that afternoon in the hospital's bathroom. According to Nick Patsidis, a midwife left them as Kathy Patsidis was going into delivery.[41]

"She's gone to the toilet," recalled Nick Patsidis, "and all of a sudden she screams and says I can't hold it and the baby's coming…"[42]

Hearing his wife in agony, to his horror, Nick Patsidis dashed into the bathroom to find her on the floor giving birth. Instinctively, he opened his wife's legs and caught the baby as she was being pushed out.[43]

"I ran into the toilet and there's my little baby girl coming out of my wife with the umbilical cord around her neck, turning blue," said Nick Patsidis.[44] "I've actually gone and grabbed [her] head from falling…"[45]

Kathy Patsidis used the call buttons in the bathroom to summon midwives.[46] When they arrived, Nick Patsidis was holding the baby.[47] Fortunately, Kathy Patsidis and the baby, Marissa, are healthy.[48]

Hospital administrators offered little compassion. "This was not a staff shortage issue. This was about a very quick birth," explained Dr. Michael Nicholl, director of maternity services at the hospital. "In a labor that from start to finish is an hour's duration it is a near impossible task... All women know that the starting of elective procedures, like inductions of labor, do depend on the activity of the ward at the time."[49]

But Nick Patsidis believed the midwives were purposefully delaying his wife's delivery. "The whole day was 'we do not have enough staff, I'm sorry we are extremely busy,'" he said. "They were prolonging it as much as they could [because] they didn't want it to happen... They [midwives] were coming and going and when things were happening they weren't able to deal with it."[50]

Maria Patsidis, Nick Patsidis' mother, went further by accusing the hospital of lying and covering up "something... out of a horror movie." She added: "It wasn't (a quick labor). The midwife who was standing on top of Kathy should have known what this was. She didn't call a doctor, she didn't call anybody."[51]

CHILD WAITS HOURS IN PAIN INSIDE HOSPITAL, ONLY TO BE SENT ELSEWHERE

Three-year-old Logan Birney was forced to wait hours in a Tenterfield, Australia hospital for doctors to attend to his bleeding mouth. Once examined, doctors gave him a mild painkiller and left his mother to take him to another, faraway hospital for follow-up treatment.[52]

One morning in late April 2008, Logan accidentally slammed his mouth into the windowsill when he jumped from his bed. The impact ripped open his gums, broke off one tooth and twisted another seven teeth. The boy's mother, Julie Birney, said she wrapped a towel over his bloody mouth and around his shoulder "like a big bib with him dribbling."

"His mouth was so swollen that he couldn't swallow saliva," Birney explained. "One tooth fell out and I had to put it back in his mouth."

They immediately set out for Prince Albert Memorial hospital in Tenterfield. When they arrived, however, the only medical attention provided was from a nurse, who took Logan's blood pressure and temperature. It would be hours before a doctor would examine Logan.

"A nurse came back in and said the doctor would be back in half an hour," Julie recalled. "I asked on the progress of the doctor one and a half hours later."

Meanwhile, the boy could not drink any water in case he needed surgery. In pain, he passed out during the tedious wait.

"I said to the nurse, I think he went into shock," Birney said. "He ended up sleeping over an hour."

Logan would have to wait until 1:40 pm to 2:15 pm, depending on reports,[53] for a doctor to see him. Logan was given merely a common pain-reliever, Panadol – similar to Tylenol – and a prescription for antibiotics. The doctor also provided a referral for an ear, nose and throat specialist – but in a different town, Lismore, roughly 100 miles away.

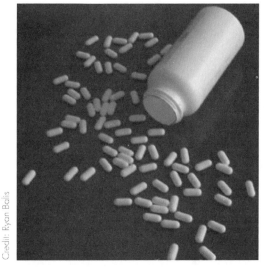

Credit: Ryan Balis

When an accident tore open the gums of 3-year-old Logan Birney, broke off one of his teeth and twisted another seven, Prince Albert Memorial hospital in Tenterfield, Australia prescribed painkillers and discharged him.

It made little sense to Birney – or the specialist's office – why Logan should go to an ear, nose and throat doctor instead of a dentist. The specialist's office told Birney Logan "would sit and wait and then be referred to someone else."

Unfortunately, the hospital's dental unit at Prince Albert Memorial was scheduled to be closed the following week. Thus, for Logan to receive necessary mouth care, Birney had to take him to a dentist nearly 60 miles away in Glen Innes and await a decision on whether his teeth would be wired or removed. Meanwhile, Logan had to manage eating only soft food.

Disturbing as Birney's experience was, he is but one of three youngsters in a two week period at Prince Albert Memorial "forced to wait hours for treatment, pain relief and a full clinical assessment," according to the Tenterfield Star. The hospital discharged all three children with Panadol, forcing the children's parents to search on their own for follow-up treatment the next day.[54]

WOMAN IN LABOR STORED IN HOSPITAL'S STOREROOM UNTIL A BED BECAME AVAILABLE

Staff at a major public hospital in Southport, Australia left a woman in labor on the floor of a hospital storeroom for several hours because no maternity beds were available.

The pregnant woman, identified only as Erica, arrived at Gold Coast Hospital at 8 am in May 2008. Though in labor, she waited in a closed waiting room for one hour until she was moved to a mattress on the floor of a linen storeroom.[55] There, with husband Mitch and sister Maurita, Erica endured an agonizing three hours waiting for a room to become available in the maternity ward.[56] She nearly gave birth before reaching a bed.[57]

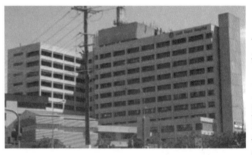

"They said they were too busy and we would have to wait for a bed and we might have to have the baby in the foyer," Erica recalled being told upon her arrival at the hospital. "The lady said 'We know how to do that and if you want to get more comfortable, get on your hands and knees… [but] I didn't feel like doing that with people walking past."[58]

Because of a bed shortage, a woman in labor was told to wait on the floor of a linen storeroom at Gold Coast Hospital in Southport, Australia.

Being stuck on the floor in cramped quarters also did not lend itself as a suitable place for doctors to monitor Erica's condition.

"She wanted pain relief but they wouldn't really give it to her because they couldn't examine her properly, so they ended up giving her the gas," explained Maurita.[59] (Dr. Adrian Nowitzke, CEO of Gold Coast Health, denied that Erica received no pain relief while in the storeroom.)[60]

The wait was particularly unpleasant because the room did not have air conditioning. Moreover, for the first 45 minutes Erica had to use spare blankets as a makeshift pillow until one was found for her.[61]

"We thought 'Stuff this, we'll look after ourselves' and pulled heaps of blankets out and tried to make it as comfortable as we could," said Maurita. "I sat on the floor next to her. It was disgusting."[62]

During the remainder of the painful wait, the family was left alone 90 percent of the time, and the family became increasingly nervous that Erica would give birth on the floor.[63]

"We started to get pretty stressed," said Maurita. "Surely there was somewhere they could take her to have a baby boy?"[64]

Eventually, roughly four hours after arriving at the hospital, a room opened and Erica was given a proper bed. She soon gave birth to a baby boy, Jackson. Despite being overjoyed and while praising the hospital staff for doing their job, Erica does not plan to have another child because of this and other distressful incidents in hospitals.[65]

"Being in a bed earlier would have saved me a lot of pain," she said. "In the storeroom you couldn't get comfortable."[66]

Dr. Nowitzke apologized personally for the mishap, but he acknowledged that the hospital might again experience such a bed shortage. "He said at the moment it might, but in the future it won't, so that's good to hear," Mitch, the husband, recalled.[67]

At the time, Gold Coast Hospital's facilities included eight delivery rooms and two alternative birth center rooms. On the day of Erica's birth, the hospital delivered 17 babies – between an additional 7-9 more than average.[68]

WAIT PROMPTS CANCER SUFFERER TO SPEND $10,000 FOR PRIVATE TREATMENT

Instead of waiting on the public care health system for six and a half weeks for urgent cancer treatment, an Australian man paid $10,000 AUD (~$8,400 USD) for immediate care at a private facility.[69]

Peter Nelson, 63, from Cairns, Queensland had terminal cancer in his spine and was in excruciating pain. Despite his dire condition, Australia's government-managed health care system would have Nelson wait seven weeks for life-extending radiation treatment at the public Townsville Hospital.

In early May 2008, Nelson faced a decision whether to wait until June 20 for publicly-provided treatment or travel to a remote private facility and pay $10,000 for immediate care.

"I think I'd have walked through the wall in sheer desperation if I had to wait," Nelson said. "But it's harder for my poor wife… to wake up and find me in tears because of the pain, she doesn't know what to do. It's just humanly unbearable sometimes."

Not able to suffer any longer, Nelson and wife, Bev, "packed [their] bags" for seven days of pain relief treatment at the Wesley Private Hospital in Brisbane.

Though his pain was relieved, Nelson regrets that other cancer patients in Queensland face major delays for urgent treatment.

"Those people believe [the government] when they say they will be treated in 20 days and they don't know it's just not true," he said.

Under health care standards in Queensland, 10 days is the maximum waiting time within which cancer patients should receive radiation treatment. But at Townsville Hospital, the average wait time was 27 days – nearly three times the allowable limit – according to a leaked government memo.

However, health officials disputed the comprehensiveness of the memo, calling the figures only a "snapshot" and its contents for planning purposes.[70]

FOUR-YEAR WAIT PROMPTS DO-IT-YOURSELF DENTISTRY

For most of us, putting up with a severe toothache for longer than a week would be too much to bear, but one Australian man languished for four years on a public waiting list for a dentist before eventually taking out his own rotten tooth himself.

Jeffrey Miners, 58, a retiree from Bega in New South Wales (NSW), desperately needed 13 teeth extracted to relieve excruciating gum pain.[71]

"I only got one decent tooth in my head, apart from the four rotten ones at the front, and the rest are just old teeth that have snapped off at the gum levels," Miners explained.[72]

Miners recalled that since 2001 he waited on various lists for dental work, receiving only "one filling done in a tooth, back in 2005, and that's in a seven-year wait." In

2004, Miners was placed on the NSW public waiting list for dental surgery. Yet, despite the intense pain in his gums, by 2008, Miners still had not moved to the top of the list to receive urgent treatment.[73]

"Nothing was being done for me, and it [the cavity] was getting to a size that it was interfering with me health," Miners explained. "Every day for two or three weeks solid prior to the extraction I was having six to eight aspirins, six to eight paradine [painkillers] for it... I was sleepless... through the nights and days and it was just agony."[74]

Miners explained that many of his teeth had decayed because of a "chemical imbalance" in his mouth. The combination of drugs he took for different health ailments produced a side effect that deteriorated his teeth.[75] And because of his bad heart, doctors needed to operate at a hospital with a cardio backup system available in case Miners suffered a heart attack.[76]

"Because... I have other medical issues, that they couldn't extract me teeth normally in a dental chair under just a local anesthetic because I have a cardiac problem," Miners said.[77]

In March 2008, Miners underwent heart bypass surgery. He recovered from the operation and was in condition to have the surgery to remove his teeth. Yet, he was told it would be another 18 months until he would receive an operation at Prince of Wales Hospital in Sydney.[78]

Living on disability income, Miners was unable to afford private dental care,[79] but the prospect of facing a seemingly unending wait on the public health care system while living with intense pain and daily painkillers that Miners said caused him to feel "like a zombie" was intolerable. In late May 2008, Miners took the extraordinary step of pulling out his own aching molar tooth.[80]

"Through inaction, I had to start taking action myself," Miners said.[81] "I kept working on it to loosen it, the cavity was so big I could fit my forefinger into it, and I just pulled it out."[82]

According to Jillian Skinner, a Member of Parliament in NSW and Shadow Health Minister, nearly 160,000 people in 2008 were on waiting lists for dental treatment in NSW,[83] Australia's most populous state.[84]

"You don't need to be a dentist to see that patients like Jeffrey Miners need urgent dental care, but the [NSW Premier Morris] Iemma Government is so incompetent it can't even get that right," Skinner charged.[85]

TEENAGER'S SEVERED FINGERS PUT ON ICE, AS WAS HIS SURGERY

An Australian teenager who severed three of his fingers in a workplace accident waited nearly two full days inside two hospitals for his fingers to be repaired.

McKenneth Atkinson, then 19, from the town of Pinjarra in the Australian state of Western Australia, was in training to become a mechanic when the accident occurred in July 2008. Atkinson was taken by ambulance to the public Royal Perth Hospital (RPH) around 3 pm on a Thursday.[86]

There was a need to treat Atkinson right away to maximize the chance he would regain usage of his fingers. Instead, he waited with the severed fingers in a bowl of ice inside the hospital's emergency department for the next 28 hours. A ward bed would need to become available before Atkinson would be moved to surgery.[87]

Colin Atkinson, the teenager's father, scolded Australia's government managed health care for the delay. "I couldn't believe how pathetic our public health system can be," he said.[88]

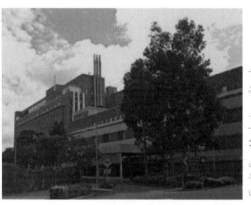

Because of a bed shortage, rather than reattach them immediately, staff at Royal Perth Hospital put McKenneth's Atkinson's three severed fingers into a bowl of ice.

The timing of reattaching fingers is crucial, according to Dr. Dave Mountain, spokesperson on emergency medicine with the Australian Medical Association. "Certainly if… there was a delay because they couldn't get him into a theatre [operating room] or a bed, that clearly would have compromised the outcome," he explained.[89]

Meanwhile, surgeons gave Atkinson and his family conflicting assessments. A surgeon told Atkinson on Friday night – over a day after his arrival at the hospital – that his fingers could not be saved and he would be dropped from the surgery list.[90]

"They told me there was no way of saving my fingers," Atkinson recalled. "One of the doctors had a look at it and went away and came back and said if they did the operation to save them there was still a risk they wouldn't be saved."[91]

However, a different surgeon told the family that the fingers could be reattached and regretted that surgery had not been performed earlier.[92] Still, that night, Atkinson received a ward bed and doctors prepped him for surgery. However, just when it appeared the operation would go forward, it was delayed yet again when, suddenly, the needs of a critically-injured patient demanded the surgeons' attention.[93]

"He had been waiting in emergency for about 28 hours before they shifted him into the hospital," said Colin Atkinson. "Then they had another trauma [victim] come in and he got pushed back into the ward."[94]

Finally, at midday on Saturday, Atkinson was transferred to Mount Private Hospital, a privately-run facility, for the operation.[95] He was discharged the following day.[96]

"The patient was not able to be moved to a ward sooner because the hospital was experiencing heavy demand for beds," said a spokesman for RPH,[97] one of Australia's largest hospitals.[98] "The hospital is sorry about Mr. Atkinson's wait for a ward bed."[99]

Despite the apology, the wait for Atkinson was extremely nerve-racking. "Basically, it was hard to come to terms with the decision the doctors made in such a short time, which I have to deal with for the rest of my life," he said.[100] "I remember feeling so helpless in the emergency department. I was angry at the state of the health system,"[101] Atkinson would later recall.

In April 2009, the Western Australia state government began requiring state emergency departments to follow a new "Four Hour Rule Program." The new regulation states that a target of "98 per cent of patients are to be seen in emergency departments and admitted, transferred or discharged within a four-hour timeframe, unless they are required to remain within the emergency department for clinical reasons."[102]

CHILD WAITS TWO YEARS FOR TONSIL REMOVAL

Melissa Williams believes the government-managed health care system in Australia has treated her six-year-old daughter, a chronic tonsillitis sufferer, as just another face among a crowd of waiting, neglected patients.[103]

Williams' daughter, Samara Cupit, suffered from chronic tonsillitis. The outbreaks and staph infections that result occur several times a week and caused Samara to miss school frequently.

"She's constantly on antibiotics and really weak and feverish and she gets a rash on her face," Williams explained at the time.

Removing Samara's tonsils is a routine operation that could have resolved the affliction immediately. But for two years, attempts by the girl's general practitioner to land an appointment for a specialist's evaluation – the first hurdle on the way to an eventual operation – were not successful.

"We've been waiting for the phone call but we've heard nothing," Williams said then. "We can't even get on a waiting list to see a doctor but after that we'd have to go on the waiting list for the operation."

Despite missing many days of her first school year, Samara did not move up the waiting list at the local Gold Coast Hospital, a public facility. Frustrated with the wait, Samara's doctor contacted a different public hospital in Ipswich, which is over 50 miles away from the family's home in Nerang, Queensland.

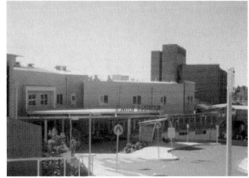

Finally, Samara was granted an appointment at Ipswich Hospital in mid-September 2008 – after two years waiting for treatment.

Six-year-old Samara Cupit waited two years for an appointment to see a specialist at Ipswich Hospital about having her tonsils removed.

Samara is perhaps one of the lucky ones, as hundreds of patients remain on the elective surgery waiting list in Australia. According to government health figures,[104] as of June 2008, some 2,786 patients were on the waiting list for elective surgery at Gold Coast Hospital. Some 440 of these patients were enduring a "long wait," which is defined as a wait longer than clinically recommended.[105]

According to the same report, when including all public hospitals in the state of Queensland, there were 34,703 patients waiting for elective surgery – 249 additional patients from July 2007. Of this total, over 7,500 were patients on the "long wait" list.[106]

ARTHRITIS SUFFERER FORCED TO WAIT NEARLY THREE YEARS FOR ANKLE SURGERY

Jennifer Haffenden of Croydon, Australia suffers from painful arthritis in her ankle. The retired 65-year-old can barely make it around to help her disabled husband and 91-year-old mother. Despite desperately needing surgery, she expects to wait nearly three years on the Australian government-managed health system.[107]

Jennifer's ankle had gradually worsened over a three-year period. By the start of 2007, the pain was unbearable. Putting any weight on it caused her to "hit the roof," requiring the use of crutches.

Jennifer had been waiting a couple of months for an appointment for corrective surgery when she received an appointment notice in the spring of 2007. Optimism turned to horror when she learned the appointment date just to see an orthopedic specialist at the public Maroondah Hospital was June 2008.

"I thought it was for this year and I nearly turned up [at the hospital] before I realized it was June 2008," Jennifer said.

By that time, her wait for a consultation would have been 14 months. On top of that wait, she likely faced an even longer 18-month wait for the eventual operation. For Jennifer, the logic of such an incredible delay when she was in obvious need of help did not make sense.

"It's very short sighted because the longer people have to wait for an operation, the worse the problem gets and the more it's going to cost," she explained.

Desperately needing surgery, Jennifer went to an orthopedic specialist as a private patient. Though the wait was less than two weeks, the cost for an operation done privately – *i.e.*, off the public health care system – was $4,000 AUD (~$3,300 USD). Instead, Jennifer opted to go on the 14-month public waiting list for the same specialist.

The wait has not been easy for Jennifer. Not only does she suffer from the arthritis in her ankle, but she also has heart ailments and Meniere's disease, which is an ear disorder causing dizziness and nausea. Moreover, she cares for her 79-year-old husband, Roy, who has had back surgery and is in a back brace. She also helps her elderly mother, who lives in a nursing home.

"It is really very difficult," Jennifer said.

AUSTRALIAN CHILDREN WAIT FOR HEART OPERATIONS

A 10-month-old was one of 400 children in Victoria, Australia waiting for cardiac surgery.[108] Julian Michielin needed an operation on his narrow arteries and for a hole in his heart. But the infant had been forced to wait through four surgery cancellations at the Royal Children's Hospital.[109]

Julian was scheduled for surgery once in July 2008 and twice more that August, but each surgery was cancelled because the hospital lacked an intensive care bed for recovery. Julian's fourth scheduled operation was cancelled yet again the day before it was supposed to take place on August 28th.[110]

"We were disappointed again with no operation," said Louisa Michielin, the baby's mother. "We weren't surprised – we knew the call was going to come."[111]

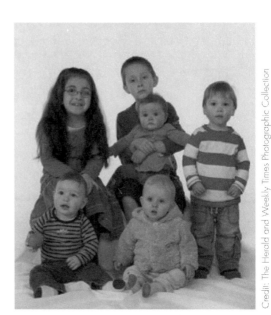

Michielin had to pay extremely close attention to Julian's condition while Julian remained on the waiting list. "[Julian] had his moment where we had to restrict him because he went blue around the mouth," she explained, "so we shifted him so he was not so active and the heart condition was taking over."[112]

"We just have to put him in the pram [stroller] and push him around so that he will stay still," Michielin added. "We just can't wait for the day where we don't have to do this – when Julian can play and sit down on his own and we know nothing will happen to him."[113]

Julian Michielin (front left) endured four cancelled heart operations at the Royal Children's Hospital in Victoria, Australia.

Credit: The Herald and Weekly Times Photographic Collection

According to Australia's Herald Sun, the Royal Children's Hospital boasts world-class heart surgeons. The hospital has a total of only 17 intensive care beds but not enough specially trained nurses required for round-the-clock monitoring.[114] Because of this, the hospital is forced to call off a significant number of operations.

Unfortunately, cancelled operations for children and babies such as Julian are common. Some 60 operations were cancelled in July 2008 alone. On one Friday in August 2008, the hospital cancelled all cardiac surgery.[115]

"We have the best surgeons you can get and they just can't do what they are supposed to be doing," said Penny Brunton, a frustrated mother of an eight-month-old whose surgery the hospital cancelled seven times in one month. Her boy, Lincoln, was booked for surgery two days after he had to be rushed to the hospital after turning blue, but that scheduled operation, the seventh, was called off.[116]

Finally, soon after the Herald Sun publicized these boys' ordeals, they and several other children waiting for heart surgery were operated on and are now healthy.[117]

GOVERNMENT GUIDELINES SAY CRUSHED HAND SHOULD BE TREATED IN EIGHT HOURS; HOSPITAL WITH WAITING LINE MAKES THAT FOUR DAYS

Following a motorcycle accident that crushed his hand and partially severed a finger, Bob Skinner waited four days for treatment in a government hospital in Australia.[118]

Bob, 39, was forced to wait in terrible pain and without a meal each day while doctors attended to other patients with conditions considered more pressing.

The accident happened in late August 2008 near Bob's home in Goodna, Australia. He was admitted to Princess Alexandra Hospital, which is one of the area's major specialist hospitals with a staff over 5,000,[119] that night, a Thursday.

Government health guidelines say Bob should have been treated within eight hours and absolutely not longer than 24 hours after admittance, but three surgery cancellations delayed an operation because hospital staff had too many patients with higher priority needs to treat Bob on schedule.

"I had two morphine shots each day for the pain," Bob said. "Every time I moved, a bolt of pain would shoot from my hand and I couldn't sleep."

What made the wait even more unbearable was Bob did not receive meals each day, apparently as a precaution in case his number was called for surgery. He ate only twice over the four days waiting in the hospital.

"Eventually I got so fed up I got them to disconnect my drip and I was over at the fast food joint across the road in my hospital gown," Bob recalled.

Finally, Bob underwent an operation on Monday, four days after being admitted. Despite subjecting Bob to an enormously painful wait, hospital staff justified the delay.

"Where it is unlikely that there will be a change in the outcome of an operation, an operation receives lower priority over one that will either save a life or improve the end outcome for the patient," explained Dr. David Thiele, clinical chief executive at Princess Alexandra. "Mr. Skinner's surgery was prioritized according to the nature of the injury and the likely outcome of surgery, which would not have changed the end result of injury, that being partial amputation of his finger."

Bob is not the only patient enduring a lengthy wait at Princess Alexandra. According to government records, thousands of other patients are on the waiting list there for surgery. As of April 1, 2009, some 4,293 patients were waiting for elective surgeries there.[120] Of this number, 1,683 patients were on the "long wait" – meaning wait times longer than clinically recommended.[121]

YOUNG MOTHER ON WAITING LIST LEFT UNABLE TO SWALLOW FOR TWO YEARS

Biljana Silke struggled each time she ate or drank.[122] At the time of her ordeal with the government-managed Australian health care system, the then-30-year-old mother of three from Noble Park North had a rare condition called achalasia. A short operation to correct the condition, which causes food and most liquids to become lodged in the esophagus, was all that was needed to make Silke's life immensely easier. Nonetheless, Silke had a long wait for relief.

For two years, Silke put up with a diet of soft and mushy foods, such as porridge and soup. She used water to force down her food, because achalasia affects the normal functioning of the esophagus, preventing esophageal muscles from relaxing to allow food and liquids to pass into the stomach.

"I never have a good meal – every single meal is a struggle," said Silke, who at the time was enduring a choking sensation whenever she tried to swallow. "I have three young children, aged 11 months, three years and 11 to look after, and can barely look after myself at the moment."

After the birth of her youngest son, Silke's discomfort increased. In December 2004, she was added to a "semi-urgent" surgery waiting list for the one-hour corrective "keyhole" operation at Monash Medical Centre, a government-managed hospital, but after four months, Silke told her surgeon she was in agony and needed the operation soon.

Silke was bumped up to an "urgent" waiting list, which meant surgery could be expected after a six-week wait. Eventually, she was booked for surgery on April 12, 2005 – only to find the operation cancelled because of a patient emergency.

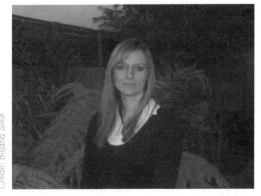

Credit: Biljana Silke

Biljana Silke waited two years for a one-hour operation to correct a condition that made it extremely difficult for her to swallow food or liquids.

Silke received a new appointment for the last week of April. The day of the scheduled surgery, Silke was told she was first in line and was prepped for surgery. However, two elderly patients requiring immediate treatment came into the hospital. Later that day, Silke was told that surgery had been postponed and possibly would be rescheduled for the next day, but with a different surgeon.

The third time was not her charm. At 11:30 am that next day, after Silke had gone without food for a considerable time, she was told the operation was yet again cancelled.

"I hadn't eaten for 24 hours; I felt weak and I felt sick and distraught," Silke recalled. "I had only had a bowl of soup and a few glasses of water in 42 hours. I almost passed out in the corridor on the way home... My children were extremely distressed about being separated from me."

Silke was told her surgery would be rescheduled within weeks. Instead, her difficulty at Monash Medical Center made headlines in the Australian press.

Two days after her story appeared in the Herald Sun, the newspaper reported that Silke had undergone successful surgery. Afterward, Silke was ecstatic about finally being able to enjoy her favorite food, doughnuts, and eat a normal meal out.[123]

"I'm just looking forward to the simple things in life and leading a happy, healthy life," she said.[124]

BABY FALLS TO HOSPITAL FLOOR IN HUMILIATING MISCARRIAGE

Amanda Booker's joy in carrying her second child turned to tragedy.[125]

17 weeks into her pregnancy, Booker's contractions were three minutes apart. The 21-year-old Barrack Heights, Australia woman rushed to Wollongong Hospital on the advice of her doctor, worried that she was suffering a miscarriage, but upon her arrival at the government-managed facility, she was told to sit in the waiting area.

"I was in agonizing pain," Amanda recalled. "I was clutching my stomach and I kept going up to the nurse saying, 'I'm really in a lot of pain – can someone please get me to a doctor?'"

After more than an hour, Amanda still had not been examined, despite pleading with the nurse. "I was sort of hushed back to my seat and told just to wait for the doctor and the doctor was coming," she said.

Finally, a nurse called her to a triage room, but while moving from the waiting area, Amanda suddenly gave birth.

"I said [to the nurse], 'something's coming out'… out came a bag and I could see my baby inside it," Amanda said. "It fell to the floor… I've never forgotten the noise it made."

What made losing her baby boy more humiliating was the door to the triage room was left open. Unfortunately, a group of men involved in a bar fight were outside the room to witness the event.

"The men [in the waiting room] stopped their mucking around and… looked quite concerned," Amanda said. "I've never seen men look compassionate before."

According to New South Wales state regulations, women suspected of suffering a miscarriage are to be moved to a maternity ward immediately. The regulations were in response to a health ministry report that investigated an 82-minute delay inside another New South Wales hospital that led to a patient, Jana Horska, suffering a miscarriage in the bathroom.[126]

"If a woman turns up and she's going to lose her baby or go into early-term labor she should be rushed immediately to the birthing unit to give birth or to lose her baby," Amanda said. "The experience of a pre-term birth is horrific enough without it being more embarrassing or demeaning."

Curiously, hospital records indicate that Amanda was moved to the triage room "immediately upon arrival."

As for Amanda, she buried her stillborn son with a clear dent on his head because he hit the hospital floor. She remains "haunted" by the incident.

BLOOD-DRENCHED WOMAN IN LABOR LOSES BABY AFTER SEVEN-HOUR WAIT FOR DOCTOR

Blood-soaked clothes and severe, stabbing labor pains are obvious signs of a troubled pregnancy. Nevertheless, 20-year-old Meagan Pringle would have to endure seven painful hours waiting in a public South African hospital before receiving medical attention, ultimately, with tragic results.[1]

On March 12, 2005, Pringle, of Kleinskool, South Africa, arrived at Dora Nginza Hospital around 1 am along with her parents. The pregnant woman's clothes were covered in blood and she was in excruciating pain. She asked to see a doctor immediately, but hospital staff told Pringle to "go and sit in the queue" with some 10 other pregnant women also waiting for treatment.

"The nurse was rude and not very sympathetic," Pringle recalled. "I was told to wait in a queue even though I was drenched in blood. I begged her to get a doctor."

Pringle became drowsy, but the nurse twice more told her to wait for a doctor. As the hours passed in the waiting hall, Pringle, increasingly agitated, went in search of a doctor herself. The hospital had only one doctor on duty that night, but Pringle managed to find an intern who examined her and moved her to the hospital's maternity department, where she continued to wait her turn.

"I was so worried," Pringle said. "I thought my son and I would die. I remember praying that nothing should happen to us..."

At 7 am, it was determined that Pringle's baby was in jeopardy. However, it would take roughly another hour for the doctor at last to attend to Pringle, just before she gave birth at 8:15 am. Tragically, though the full-term baby, named Vince, was otherwise healthy, he could not breathe. He later was pronounced dead.

"[M]y worst fear was realized when they told me he had died," Pringle said. "I looked at his little dead body in the labor ward. My heart was filled with pain."

Following the death of her newborn, Pringle sued the Eastern Cape Health Department and the hospital's medical superintendent for negligence. In March 2008, Judge Johan Froneman of the Port Elizabeth High Court awarded Pringle a R200,000 (~$25,600 USD) judgment. Judge Froneman ruled that if hospital staff had monitored the baby more closely, a caesarian section could have been performed and Vince would have lived.

Pringle told the court she continued to suffer immensely over her loss. She described the day Vince died as "the worst day of my life."

"Although I have another daughter, Michaela, I am still struggling to piece my life back together," she said. "I did not sue for money. I sued them so they could better the circumstances for other women who have to make use of the public health care system."

"Nobody deserves to go through this sort of trauma," Pringle added.

The Dora Nginza Hospital made headlines in 2007 when a government health official warned that severe short-staffing put the hospital in "a crisis."[2] Fred Rank, head of clinical governance for Port Elizabeth's hospitals, reported that only one nurse was available for every 90 patients. He emphasized that the hospital was so understaffed that doctors and nurses were forced to do extra duty as hospital cleaners and baggage carriers.[3]

"In the casualty ward we have two nurses attending to about 30 patients. In the maternity ward two or three midwives attend to about 10 women [in labor] at any time," Rank told the National Council of Provinces, the upper house of South Africa's legislature.[4]

TWO HOSPITALS FAIL TO TREAT FIVE-YEAR-OLD AFTER MAJOR CAR CRASH

A five-year-old South African girl involved in a major car accident died after 10 hours of being shuffled among three different hospitals without treatment.[5]

One evening in May 2008, Munashe Princess, 5, was traveling with her stepmother, Judith Tshipugu, and father, Ezekiël Keswa, originally of Zimbabwe. The family was moving its belongings to the town of Kwaggafontein to escape violence in Duduza. Tragically, however, the stepmother and daughter, riding in a separate car, were injured when they struck another vehicle head-on.

"I was driving in a bakkie [pickup truck] behind the car," explained Keswa, the girl's father. "Tshipugu swerved to the right because a car had suddenly stopped and they were in a head-on collision right in front of me."

Seeing his daughter in so much pain was "terrible to see," said Keswa. "My daughter was trapped in the wreckage and I could hear her crying."

Rescue workers had to free Munashe from the car using the rescue tool jaws of life. Along with her stepmother, Munashe was taken to Delmas Hospital with broken bones and chest trauma for what should have been immediate medical treatment. What ensued was a 10-hour ordeal that took the family from one hospital to the next.

Keswa said his daughter "called to me and insisted that I stay with her." He added, "She asked me for water, but the doctors said she couldn't take in anything because she might go to theatre [operating room]."

Doctors at Delmas Hospital were the first to bump Munashe to a different hospital. Despite Munashe's serious condition possibly requiring surgery, both stepmother and daughter were transferred to Witbank Hospital, a specialist hospital.

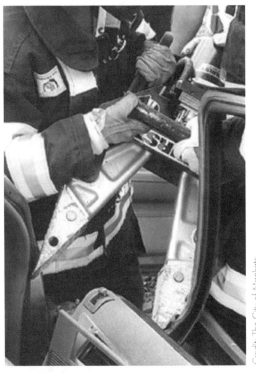

Though rescue workers released 5-year-old Munashe Princess from a smashed car (model shown), she died after a 10-hour ordeal in which her family went from one hospital to another hoping to receive treatment.

Keswa followed them to Witbank Hospital in his car, arriving roughly four hours after the accident. Upon his arrival, he discovered his family seemingly neglected.

"When I got there at about 22:00, they were still in casualty [emergency department]. To one side a nurse was sitting and sleeping," he recalled.

At roughly midnight, doctors told Keswa that the hospital did not have the necessary equipment working to operate on his daughter. Yet again, Munashe would need to be transferred.

But it took roughly two hours for an ambulance to arrive. To make the situation worse, the ambulance first needed to return to Delmas to switch drivers before taking Munashe, her father and stepmother to what was their third medical destination.

"I sat alone in the back of the ambulance with my wife and my daughter," said Keswa. "The nurse was in the front with the driver."

Now back at Delmas Hospital, the ambulance sat in the parking lot for 30 minutes. Frustrated, Keswa went inside the hospital to inquire about the delay.

"I went in to hear where they were," said Keswa. "They said they were busy."

Finally, the ambulance left with the family to Pretoria Academic Hospital. According to an account in the South African daily newspaper, Beeld, several elite specialists had assembled there to attempt to save the girl's life. However, by the time the ambulance arrived at 4 am, it was too late for Munashe. She died of chest trauma.

"My daughter was the best thing ever. I saw her suffering," said Keswa. "I'm trying to handle it, but it is unbelievably difficult."

As for Keswa's wife, she remained in the hospital. An official investigation into Munashe's death was undertaken by local health authorities. Moreover, the South African Human Rights Commission, an independent institution, was asked to determine if human rights violations occurred.[6]

GOVERNMENT HEALTH OFFICIAL SAYS WOMAN IN LABOR'S FRANTIC SEARCH FOR EMERGENCY ROOM "NOT AN EMERGENCY"

A young South African woman feared her pregnancy would end in miscarriage when two government hospitals did not have either staff or facilities available to treat her the day she went into labor. After waiting hours without help, the woman and her family frantically rushed over 60 miles to a third hospital just in time to deliver the baby.

Sina Minnie, 21, of Middelburg, South Africa went into labor early one morning in July 2008. Her husband called for an ambulance to take Minnie to Middelburg Hospital, the town's local public hospital. However, the ambulance did not arrive for more than two hours.[7]

Minnie nonetheless managed to get to Middelburg Hospital that morning, but there she waited nearly four hours without receiving any medical attention. The family was told to wait because the hospital had "only cleaners" on duty at the time. Eventually, the couple decided to find a different hospital.

At 11 am, the couple arrived at Witbank Hospital, another government facility, but, yet again, there was a delay getting her into a delivery room.

"I was told that they didn't have any beds available and that I should just stand and wait in the passage," Minnie said. "The pain was unbearable."

The family waited an hour and a half at Witbank before realizing they needed to find Minnie another hospital – one with a delivery room available – and quickly. Delivery was imminent. Minnie's father-in-law, Frans Nagel, rushed her to yet another government hospital in Ermelo, over 60 miles away.

"I'm going to lose my child!" Minnie screamed anxiously in transit. "My father-in-law wanted to know if I could hold on so that he could drive me to Ermelo 100km away."

But the baby could no longer wait. Only a few miles from the hospital, his "head and shoulders were already coming out," Minnie recalled. Almost immediately after arriving at Ermelo Hospital, Minnie gave birth to a son, named Schalk, born roughly one month prematurely.

Following the birth, Minnie developed an infection that required medical attention. The family initiated a legal challenge against the government's health care service.

Minnie's ordeal drew little sympathy from Fish Mahalela, then the Mpumalanga Department of Health and Social Development MEC – that is, Member of the Executive Council, a cabinet-level department at the provincial level. "It was not an [emergency]," declared Mahalela, who laughed at the story, "because, if it was an [emergency], the patient could have delivered on the floor."[8]

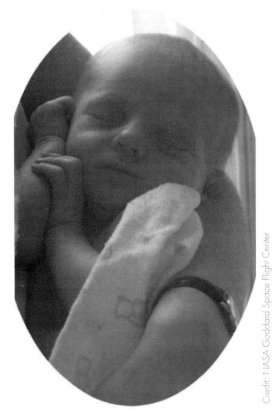

Credit: NASA Goddard Space Flight Center

In labor, Sina Minnie went to three hospitals before finding one with a delivery room available. Her son (model shown) was half-born by the time she was finally admitted.

NURSES LEAVE MOM TO GIVE BIRTH ALONE IN DIRTY HOSPITAL BATHROOM, THEN SCOLD HER FOR NOT GIVING BIRTH AT HOME

A 32-year-old South African woman gave an account of her horrific childbirth at Mapulaneng Hospital, a government-managed facility in Bushbuckridge, South Africa. While she was vomiting and in labor, the woman reports, rude nurses left her to give birth on a bathroom floor, despite her cries for help.[9]

Following her ordeal, the mother, Nikie Judith Mashego, provided details of her experience to hospital officials.

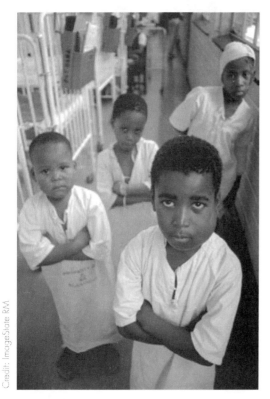

Having a child in a South African public hospital can be a harrowing experience.

Credit: ImageState RM

According to a press report on Mashego's written account, she arrived at the hospital at 4 am September 21, 2008. A nurse saw her at 5:15 that morning but not again until 8 am. Mashego alleges that nurses insisted she was not due to deliver.

Meanwhile, Mashego became sick while waiting on a bench. A nurse told her to go vomit in the toilet and offered little assistance.

"The nurse told me to clean up my mess with a piece of a linen that was wet from having been used on another patient," Mashego said. "Another nurse ordered me to lie down when I cried for help."

But Mashego fell ill once again. She went to the bathroom when, suddenly, her water broke. Mashego said she cried for help but alleges the nurses did not assist her. Instead, she was left to deliver a baby boy on the floor of the bathroom.

Mashego said she pleaded for the nurses again while in the bathroom with her baby still attached. Finally, a nurse came, but would not enter the dirty bathroom. She threw Mashego a bed sheet to wrap up her baby. Astonishingly, Mashego recalled, the abusive nurse then scolded her for coming to the hospital for the delivery.

"An angry nurse asked me why I had not given birth at home since I was able to deliver on my own," Mashego reported. "I handed my baby to the nurse, who cut the umbilical cord before asking me why I could not take the placenta out since I was able to deliver without help."

Mashego's ordeal is being investigated.

"The patient has made a presentation to the hospital management and if her allegations are true her rights as a patient were violated," said Mpho Gabashane, spokesman for the Mpumalanga provincial health department.

FOURTEEN HOSPITALS TURN AWAY CRITICALLY-INJURED ELDERLY MAN

Rescue workers in Japan called 14 hospitals before finding one that would take an elderly bicyclist who collided with a motorcycle.[1]

The accident, which occurred at 10:15 pm in the Japanese city of Itami, left the 69-year-old bicyclist, who was not identified, in critical condition with back and head injuries. Paramedics arrived on the scene five minutes after the crash and administered first aid. Yet, for about an hour, they were unsuccessful at locating a hospital to treat the man.

Helpless, the elderly man waited in the ambulance at the accident scene as hospital after hospital rejected treating him, citing unavailable beds, staff shortages and a lack of equipment and specialists. All told, 14 hospitals in the neighboring prefectures – *i.e.*, governing districts – of Hyogo and Osaka refused his entry.

"There were four other emergency calls in the same time frame of that night," explained Mitsuhisa Ikemoto, the fire department spokesman. "[A]s a result, we were unable to find a hospital."

It took a second round of calls for rescue workers to find a hospital. Finally, at 11:30 that night – 75 minutes after the accident – they took him to a hospital in Itami, which had initially declined to accept him. Unfortunately, it soon became apparent that the hospital's resources that night were unsatisfactory.

At the time of his arrival at the hospital, the elderly man was already in critical condition from the accident and post-accident delay. When his condition suddenly deteriorated, hospital staff scrambled "to transfer him for better treatment," according to the Associated Press.

Two hospitals rejected that transfer request. By the time a third hospital agreed to take the man, his condition was too poor to permit him to be moved.

He died of hemorrhagic shock at about 1:15 the next morning.

The Associated Press reported that the man "initially showed stable vital signs," and, attributing the assessment to Ikemoto, reported the man "might have survived if a hospital accepted him more quickly." Ikemoto was quoted saying, "I wish hospitals are more willing to take patients..."

Rescue workers also had trouble finding a hospital to treat a 29-year-old motorcyclist who also had been involved in the crash. Despite the motorcyclist's severe injuries, the first two hospitals contacted refused to admit him. The third try succeeded, and the man was taken to a university hospital in Hyogo. Fortunately, two weeks after the accident, he was recovering.

The frustrating, and in one case, tragic experiences of the two accident victims initially denied medical care are not unique in Japan's universal health insurance system.

According to a government survey conducted by the country's Fire and Disaster Management Agency, Japanese hospitals denied admission to some 14,387 emergency patients in 2007. All 14,000-plus patients identified on paramedics' reports were rejected at least three times. Moreover, at least 3.5 percent of these victims had serious conditions, which the survey defined as requiring more than three weeks of hospitalization.[2]

PREGNANT JAPANESE WOMAN DIES AFTER EIGHTEEN HOSPITALS REJECT HER

Mika Takasaki fell into a coma while in labor but before delivering her baby. The town-run hospital in Oyodo, Japan to which she was initially admitted was unable to handle her condition. Yet, Takasaki was not whisked to another facility, because 18 hospitals declined to accept her.[3]

Takasaki was 41 weeks pregnant[4] when she was taken to Oyodocho Municipal Hospital at about 6 pm, suffering a headache.[5] Her limbs started to stiffen,[6] and she fell unconscious at about 12:15 am.[7]

The doctor initially believed Takasaki had fainted because of birthing pains, and did not believe she was suffering from a serious brain ailment.[8] However, a brain scan was not performed, despite one doctor raising the possibility of a serious issue.[9]

When Takasaki's condition deteriorated, the doctor diagnosed Takasaki with eclampsia – a dangerous complication. The doctor began to look for a hospital equipped to treat her.[10] Government data in Nara Prefecture (a regional governing district) show that some 30 percent of pregnant women needing emergency treatment are transferred to a better-equipped facility outside the district.[11]

However, 18 medical facilities turned down the transfer order. The first two hospitals contacted cited a lack of intensive care beds for a newborn. Finally, over four hours after Takasaki fell into a coma, the government-run National Cardiovascular Center one hour away in Osaka accepted Takasaki.[12]

After Mika Takasaki fell into a coma while in labor, 18 hospitals refused to admit her. When the National Cardiovascular Center in Osaka (pictured) admitted her, it became clear she had suffered a stroke.

Credit: lignis at en.wikipedia

Takasaki arrived at the hospital at 6 am, at which time doctors became aware that she had suffered a stroke.[13] Takasaki underwent emergency surgery for bleeding of the brain and her baby was delivered through a Caesarean section. However, Takasaki never regained consciousness and, tragically, passed away eight days later.[14] The baby boy, Sota, was delivered in good health.[15]

"My wife died without seeing and holding her own baby," said husband Shinsuke Takasaki. "I really urge… improvements in transport system for pregnant women so that this kind of tragedy will never be repeated."[16]

FIFTH TIME'S THE CHARM IN THE RUSSIAN HEALTH CARE BUREAUCRACY

In many American towns and cities, teenagers (and some adults, to be sure) camp out all night, if not longer, in front of electronics stores to be among the first to have the newest and hottest iPod or video game console.[1]

Life is similar in St. Petersburg, Russia – but with a dangerous twist. There the sick, elderly and handicapped can be seen spending all night waiting in extreme cold for a government-issued medical form – the first of many hurdles to getting taxpayer provided advanced medical treatment.

One such case that drew considerable media attention in Russia involved the disabled mother of a Russian blogger identified only by her Internet name, "Lassi." For Lassi's mother, it took five trips waiting outside a local administrative health center, in frigid conditions, without anything warm to drink or a toilet, just to get the referral form she needed to schedule a surgery on a bad leg.

Lassi's mother's hurt her leg in February 2006. She was taken by ambulance to the St. Petersburg State City Hospital No. 26, but was not issued a room. She instead stayed overnight in the hallway, as the cost for a room was 2,500 rubles (~$80) per day.

She was discharged, but the pain became so overpowering that eventually she could no longer stand. By March 2008, she decided to go on her own to have her leg checked further.

Unfortunately, the process for obtaining advanced medical treatment on the public health system involves spending considerable effort navigating the local bureaucracy before the patient even enters the surgery room. The first step for Lassi's mother, a retiree, was to apply for a "quota," or medical referral document, from a physician in her local health bureau. These papers – essentially rationed on a first-come, first-served basis – act as a 'pre-approval' document.

In one "oblast," or administrative region, of St. Petersburg, there is only one such health office to allocate the quotas. They are distributed once per week on Wednesdays from 10 am until 12 pm, and there is not a procedure for patients to sign up ahead of time.

As a result, nearly 100 sick people or their line-stander camp out in front of the

Orthopedic Trauma Medical Center in the cold early morning hours. Because some people wait 12 hours in line, relatives and friends of the sick take turns holding a spot.

"[P]eople in wheelchairs and on crutches, as well as their relatives and friends, start coming to that courtyard to secure their place in the waiting line from 2:30 am," reported Lassi.

But on four occasions her mother did not reach the front of the line. Lassi became involved on the fifth attempt when she learned of her mother's efforts.

"She 'was afraid to disturb me,'" Lassi recalled her mother saying. "She just tried to do it by herself. And failed."

The morning of the fifth attempt, Lassi asked friends to hold a spot in line until she arrived at 4 to 5 am. She described the scene at the health center:

> Wearing a winter coat at 5 am I was not able to be even one of the first 30 people. People are standing in a dark yard on crutches, in wheelchairs. They all recognize each other – the referral is one-time use only – and it's not the first time they don't get it. There are tons of cars. People help each other like during the blockade [of Leningrad in World War II]. [T]hey allow others to sit in relatives' cars to get warmed up. It's cold, dark, there are no bathrooms, [and] people are barely standing.

At 8:30 am, Lassi's mother arrived to take her spot in line. When the doors of the center opened at 10, she could move inside, but there were seats for only 10 people in the crowded hallway.

Finally, she obtained the referral form at 11:50 – 10 minutes before the health office closed. She is one of about 40 to 50 patients who usually receive a quota out of the 100.

However, obtaining the medical referral form was just the first step. Next, Lassi's mother was told to register the form at the "other end of the city, [and] wait in another enormous line from 1 to 5 pm to get a registration number for their form," recalled Lassi.

Unfortunately, despite a quota and registration number, the mother will continue to have to wait for a surgery date. The type she requires on her bad leg has a two-year wait.

However, following media exposure of the handicapped and elderly patients enduring overnight vigils, the local health office changed its policies and hours of operation. It now will remain open until the evening, and every patient in line will be seen. A second doctor and an additional examination room were also added.

"For me to stand here [waiting in the health center] is a real insult," said Ershova Tamara Grigoryevna, another patient in line who worked 40 years as a surgeon. "I was working during the Soviet time and could not imagine that such [a] thing would be possible. Even during the blockade [of Leningrad] we were standing in line for bread in warmth... [L]ife seemed a lot happier."

PRIME MINISTER'S LONG WAIT FOR SURGERY TYPIFIES THE HEALTH CARE EXPERIENCE IN SWEDEN

The thought of waiting in pain in an effort to score a political point would have most of us scratching our heads. But Sweden's then-Prime Minister, Göran Persson, appeared to do exactly that when he declined to obtain private treatment for an ailing hip. Instead, he took a number and waited over eight months for surgery on the Swedish government health system.

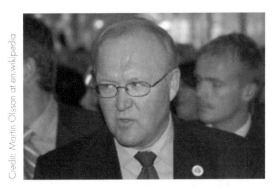

Credit: Martin Olsson at en.wikipedia

Then-Prime Minster Göran Persson's long wait for surgery is a common experience in Sweden's public health system.

Persson's well-publicized health trouble started in September 2003, when he was diagnosed with hip arthrosis. Doctors told Persson, who served as head of the Swedish Social Democratic Party from 1996 to 2007, that he needed urgent hip replacement surgery.[1]

Unfortunately for Persson, an estimated 5,000 other Swedes were already on the waiting list for the same operation. Though hip replacement surgery typically takes under two hours to complete,[2] Persson was told he would need to wait until before Christmas – that is, Christmas the following year.[3]

At the time, a privately-performed hip replacement would cost about €8,000 euros (~$11,500) and likely would be scheduled in a matter of weeks, but Persson stubbornly refused to forgo the government-managed health care system, deciding he would wait it out for his country's eventual care.[4]

"Right now I'm in quite a lot of pain, but that's not the fault of the health system," said Persson at the time. "I'm counting that this will be managed through public health care. I would be very surprised if not."[5]

During the months of waiting, Persson walked with an obvious limp and was rumored to be on strong painkillers. In 2004, he canceled an official trip to the EU-Latin America meeting held in Mexico because his hip was too bad to handle a long flight.[6]

Though his operation was scheduled for December 2004, Persson got his operation early. After an over eight-month wait,[7] he was operated on successfully in June 2004 at the public Söder Hospital in Stockholm.[8] Though he waited in pain, a

Reuters report noted that Persson may have achieved his own small victory: "[I]n a country famed for its cradle-to-grave welfare state and where politicians see themselves as ordinary folk... Swedes are likely to applaud their leader, whose party pledges 'people before markets...'"[9]

Nevertheless, Persson's wait highlights deeper problems in Sweden's government-managed health care system. A 2003 report by the Swedish National Board of Health and Welfare, a government agency, showed that only 40 percent of hip replacement patients received treatment within a three-month target period during the first four months of 2003, just prior to Persson going on the waiting list for surgery.[10]

"The main problem with Swedish health care is not its quality, but its accessibility," says Waldemar Ingdahl, director of the Stockholm-based think tank, Eudoxa.[11]

In 2007, David Hogberg, Ph.D. wrote for the National Center for Public Policy Research:

> A recent study that examined over 5,800 Swedish patients on a wait list for heart surgery found that the long wait has consequences far worse than pain, anxiety or monetary cost. In this study, the median wait time was found to be 55 days. While on the waiting list, 77 patients died. The authors' statistical analysis led them to conclude that the "risk of death increases significantly with waiting time." Another study found a mean wait time of 55 days for heart surgery in Sweden and a similar rate of mortality for those on the waiting list. Finally, a study in the Swedish medical journal Lakartidningen found that reducing waiting times reduced the heart surgery mortality rate from seven percent to just under three percent.[12]

Writing in the Journal of American Physicians and Surgeons in 2008, Sven R. Larson, Ph.D., provided real-life examples of the human cost of Sweden's rationing:

> In October 2003 Mrs. A., who lives in Malmo, Sweden, gave birth to a baby boy. She was signed out from the hospital after delivering the baby. There are not enough beds, so delivering a baby "without complications" is an outpatient procedure. Budget cuts have eliminated beds and medical staff.
>
> The next day Mr. and Mrs. A. noticed that their baby was weak and did not want to eat. As is common in Sweden, they did not call a doctor. Instead they called the tax-paid "TeleMedicine" service. Nobody advised them to go see a doctor right away.

The following day their baby died of pneumonia.

In May 2006 another couple lost their three-year-old son to the budget-starved medical system. When Mr. and Mrs. B.'s son suffered from diarrhea and had been vomiting for almost two days, they took him to the emergency room at the nearby university hospital. A doctor ordered a supply of intravenous fluids, and the boy was sent on to the pediatric clinic to have them administered. When he arrived, the nurses had no time for him. Mr. and Mrs. B. repeatedly called on the medical staff to ask why nobody was coming to give their son the intravenous fluids he so desperately needed. Every time they got the same answer: nobody has time. They have too many patients and too little staff.

Six hours later the three-year-old boy died of heart failure.

You do not have to be a child to die from denial of care in Sweden. In April 2005 Mr. C., 61 years old, became concerned about an unusual feeling of fatigue. He went to see a doctor at the local government-run clinic. The doctor sent him home with some encouraging words.

Mr. C. came back a while later with worsened symptoms. Again he was sent home after a superficial examination and with more reassurance.

Over the next year and a half Mr. C. visited this tax-paid local clinic a total of 14 times. He had no choice – all Swedes have to go through a government-run primary care physician at a tax-paid clinic in order to see a specialist. He developed blood in his urine. But the doctors refused even to take a blood test.

They told Mr. C. and his son that they were denying him the blood test because of budget restrictions imposed by government bureaucrats.

When, finally, Mr. C.'s son convinced the doctors to do one blood test, they found out that Mr. C. had cancer. He was referred to a regional hospital. There they established that his cancer, originally curable, had spread throughout his body.

There was nothing left to do. He died shortly after.[13]

Dr. Larson goes on to write of the single clinic that is open to serve the residents of Sweden's third-largest clinic. It employs security guards. As Larson writes, "The security guards serve two functions. They keep patients from becoming unruly as they sit and wait for hours to see a doctor, and they keep new patients from entering the center when the waiting room is considered full."[14]

In October 2007, the Cancerfonden, the Swedish Cancer Society, reported that the shortage of radiologists and mammography nurses in Sweden "is so serious that, if nothing is done, within a few years it will not be possible to provide mammography for women in most counties in Sweden." The group further reported that throughout the entire country, only six chest radiologists were being trained, while the average age of working mammography personnel at the time was over 50.[15]

COLON CANCER SYMPTOM? THE LINE FOR A COLONOSCOPY LASTS TWO YEARS

Sixty-one-year-old New Zealander John White could have waited two years for an urgent colon cancer test – that is, had he stuck with New Zealand's government-managed health care. Instead, White opted for private care and was treated within months.[1]

In May 2005, White visited his general practitioner after noticing blood in his stools. Because White's younger brother had been treated for colon cancer, White had an urgent need to be tested for the deadly cancer.

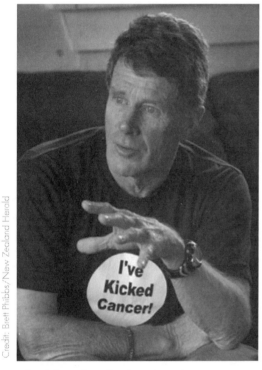

Credit: Brett Phibbs/New Zealand Herald

After John White developed a colon cancer symptom, New Zealand's public health service told him to wait two years for a colonoscopy.

Moreover, according to research conducted at the University of Otago, New Zealand has an especially high rate of colorectal cancer. 1,140 – or slightly less than half of men and women diagnosed – die because of it each year in New Zealand.[2] Early detection is key for fighting the cancer, and, as such, the New Zealand government is considering a mass-screening program.[3]

New Zealand government guidelines recommended a colonoscopy exam be administered within eight weeks for those displaying characteristic symptoms, but the need for testing White quickly seemed to be lost on public health authorities.

White's doctor referred him to Auckland City Hospital, located in the largest city in New Zealand, for a colonoscopy. But after 14 months of waiting for a scheduled test, all the while worrying that he may have life-threatening cancer, White opted to have a test done privately.

"If I had waited any longer, I know I would have died," White said. Prudently, he carried private health insurance – beyond that supposedly provided publicly – that would cover private treatment.

In July 2006, a private surgeon carried out a colonoscopy. The test showed colon cancer had spread to his lymph nodes, and an operation was scheduled at Mercy Hospital.

The following September, surgeons removed cancer from sections of the intestine and lymph nodes and followed up with chemotherapy. Since the treatment, two CT scans showed no further evidence of cancer.

In May 2007 – two years after he initially consulted a doctor in the public system – Auckland City Hospital at last got around to scheduling White for a colonoscopy.

MOTHER LEARNS A LESSON ABOUT STATE HOSPITAL CARE

In November 2008, Jordann Beckett, 3, crushed his finger in a folding camp bed. The mangled finger was deeply cut above the first joint, and only a flap of flesh kept it attached. But young Jordann didn't receive prompt surgery. Instead, his finger was bound with adhesive bandages, and he was sent home.[4]

When Jordann and his mother, Kirstian Beckett, arrived at Oamaru Hospital, a government-managed facility in Oamaru, New Zealand, an X-ray showed a broken bone at the tip of the finger. Surgery would be required to reattach the fingertip, but staff said the hospital lacked the capability to perform the operation. The boy was advised to travel to a different state hospital, Timaru Hospital.

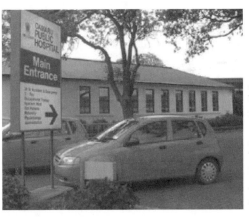

An hour later, the transfer offer was canceled. Instead, Jordann's finger was taped together with adhesive butterfly strips, and Jordann was sent home with a prescription for antibiotics and Paracetamol, which is similar to Tylenol, was recommended for the pain.

Only a flap of flesh kept 3-year-old Jordann Beckett's finger attached to his hand, but staff at Oamaru Hospital in New Zealand refused him surgery to repair it.

"The doctor didn't really care and the nurses were rough on it when they were putting the butterfly stitches on and wrapping it up," Beckett said.

Staff told Beckett to bring Jordann back in two days. The mother, angered, believed hospital staff accepted the possibility that the fingertip would be lost.

"Basically they don't care if his finger stays on or falls off," said Beckett, who accused the staff of treating her son uncaringly. "They said you can't do much about it."

But for Beckett, it was unconscionable not to try every avenue to get Jordann the surgery he needed. The following day she and Jordann made the over three-hour journey to Christchurch Hospital, a private facility.

There, Jordann's hand was X-rayed and a hand surgeon was called in to operate. The surgeon realigned the bone, removed the fingernail and stitched up the finger with thread.

Though thankful her son's sliced finger was repaired, Beckett is upset over the lack of care at the state facilities.

"I was angry," she said. "Jordann's three and a half. Who's to say he doesn't need the tip of his finger when he's grown up."

WAITING LIST AND HALF-COMPLETED SURGERY LEAVE WOMAN INFERTILE AND IN PAIN FOR 18 MONTHS

Amy Galbraith never expected to need to go under the knife twice because surgeons did not finish the job the first time.[5]

The 28-year-old Christchurch, New Zealand woman had waited a year for gynecological surgery. She needed a cyst removed from her fallopian tubes and possibly treatment for endometriosis (an external growth of the tissue lining the uterus that can result in infertility)[6] as well, if detected during the operation.

Before surgery, she was told that both the cyst and, if need be, any endometriosis adhesions would be removed during the same operation.

In mid-September 2008, Amy underwent surgery under a general anesthetic at the government-managed Christchurch Women's Hospital. She was the last patient scheduled for the day. But the anesthetist had to leave the hospital by 5:30 pm, which, Amy said, cut short the full operation. When Amy awoke, she learned that only the cyst had been removed, despite the endometriosis that was present.

"I'm really angry about being misled about what could happen," Amy said. "If you started bleeding on the table or something had gone wrong they wouldn't have just left you there, would they?"

Amy was told that she would need to undergo a second surgery to remove her grade two endometriosis. However, the wait for the second half of surgery is at least six months. The delay puts on hold the plans Amy and her partner, Bryan Riddle, have to start a family. Furthermore, the endometriosis causes lower abdominal pain and painful menstruation.

Mark Leggett, General Manager for Medical and Surgical Services at Christchurch Women's Hospital, said the surgery was not halted because the anesthesiologist needed to leave the hospital. Moreover, according to Leggett and the Canterbury District Health Board, the regional government health care provider, it is not uncommon to divide an operation into multiple sessions if it runs over.

But for Amy, the explanation is little comfort. The endometriosis causes lower abdominal pain and painful menstruation. She doesn't believe the wait for complete treatment for her condition should stretch to a year and a half.

MAN WITH SUSPECTED STROKE LEFT OVERNIGHT IN A LA-Z-BOY

Michael Wigmore never imagined he would spend the night in a recliner chair at a New Zealand hospital's emergency center while suffering what he suspected was a stroke.[7]

Wigmore, 34, called for an ambulance one afternoon in September 2008, after his right side became numb. Suspecting a stroke, Wigmore was dropped off at the government-managed Waitakere Hospital at roughly 2 pm that afternoon. He was taken in for initial tests, but the staff determined he should be transferred to a different, larger hospital to undergo further scans.

An ambulance took five-and-a-half hours to arrive for the transfer in the early morning hours. It dropped off Wigmore at North Shore Hospital – also a government-managed hospital – at 2 am.

But North Shore Hospital had no room. Staff gave Wigmore the option of sleeping in a bed parked in a corridor or in a La-Z-Boy recliner chair in a TV waiting room, which he chose.

"I thought it was kinda strange," Wigmore recalled thinking. "No one should have to sleep in a La-Z-Boy chair in a hospital. That's just a joke."

"If you have a stroke you'd like to think you can lie down somewhere and be plugged into a machine," added Wigmore's brother, Terry Hollands.

Wigmore spent about eight hours in the recliner before being put into a proper bed for further evaluation of his condition.

North Shore Hospital is investigating the matter. "The District Health Board's chief medical officer has acknowledged Mr. Wigmore's concerns and will discuss this complaint with the staff who were on duty at the time," read a hospital statement.

Wigmore's experience, while unfortunate, could have been worse. Waiting lists for surgery or to see a specialist in New Zealand's public system are commonplace and growing. While the precise number of people on waiting lists is subject to debate, present estimates range between 70,000-110,000.

PREFACE

1   Karol Sikora, "Cancer Survival in Britain," British Medical Journal, August 21, 1999, as cited by John C. Goodman, Gerald L. Musgrave and Devon M. Herrick in "Lives at Risk: Single-Payer National Health Insurance Around the World," Rowan & Littlefield Publishers/National Center for Policy Analysis, 2004, page 73.

2   Nigel Hawkes, "Patients Put at Risk by Delays in Cancer Care," Times (UK), April 3, 2007, downloaded from http://timesonline.co.uk/tol/life_and_style/health/article1605142.ece on August 10, 2009.

3   "Surgeons Blast Cancer Hold-Ups That Can Kill," London Evening Standard, March 24, 2007, available online at   http://www.thisislondon.co.uk/news/article-23386773-details/Surgeons%20blast%20cancer%20hold-ups%20that%20 can%20kill/article.do as of August 22, 2009.

4   Julian Gavaghan, "NHS is Critical," People (UK), March 4, 2007, available at http://www.people.co.uk/news/ tm_headline=nhs-is-critical--&method=full&objectid=18704339&siteid=93463-name_page.html as of August 12, 2009.

5   Julian Gavaghan, "NHS is Critical," People (UK), March 4, 2007, available at http://www.people.co.uk/news/ tm_headline=nhs-is-critical--&method=full&objectid=18704339&siteid=93463-name_page.html as of August 12, 2009.

6   Nigel Hawkes, "£35,000-a-year kidney cancer drugs too costly for NHS," Times (UK), downloaded from http:// www.timesonline.co.uk/tol/life_and_style/health/article4474425.ece on August 10, 2009.

7   "Kidney Cancer Victims Denied 'Wonder Drugs'," Sunday Times (UK), February 25, 2007, as reprinted on the website of the James Whale Fund for Kidney Cancer, downloaded from http://www.jameswhalefund.org/KidneyCancerNews_SundayTimes.html on August 10, 2009.

8   IHS Global Insight, "NICE Rebuffs Kidney Cancer Drugs for Second Time Despite Offers of Price-Sharing Agreements," downloaded from http://www.globalinsight.com/SDA/SDADetail15874.htm on August 10, 2009.

9   David Rose, "Cancer Patients Denied Life Saving 'Near Label' Drugs," Times (UK), August 14, 2009, downloaded from http://www.timesonline.co.uk/tol/life_and_style/health/article6796234.ece on ugust 14, 2009.

10   Scott Burgess-Thunderer, "Shamen on the NHS, It's Away With the Fairies," London Times, March 5, 2007, downloaded from http://timesonline.co.uk/tol/comment/columnists/guest_contributors/article1469961.ece on August 10, 2009.

11   Ed West, "Let's Get Rid of NHS Chaplains – And Boob Jobs," Telegraph (UK), April 8, 2009, downloaded from http://blogs.telegraph.co.uk/news/edwest/9424607/Lets_get_rid_of_NHS_chaplains__and_boob_jobs/ on August 10, 2009.

12   "Level of Abortions Reaches Record High of 200,000 a Year," London Evening Standard, June 19, 2007, downloaded from http://www.thisislondon.co.uk/news/article-23401185-details/Level+of+abortions+reaches+record+high+of+20 0,000+a+year/article.do on August 9, 2009.

13   Stephanie Condron, " Sex Change Ops on the NHS Have Trebled... Since the Procedure Became a 'Right,'" Daily Mail (UK), June 28, 2009, downloaded from http://www.dailymail.co.uk/health/article-1196024/Sex-change-ops-NHS-trebled--procedure-right.html on August 10, 2009.

14   John C. Goodman, Gerald L. Musgrave and Devon M. Herrick in "Lives at Risk: Single-Payer National Health Insurance Around the World," Rowan & Littlefield Publishers/National Center for Policy Analysis, 2004, page 73.

15   "Obama's Senior Moment," Wall Street Journal, August 14, 2009, downloaded from http://online.wsj.com/article/ SB10001424052970203863204574344900152168372.html on August 14, 2009.

16   "Increased Spending Not Helping," National Center for Policy Analysis, March 13, 2007, summarizing the findings of a report by the Fraser Institute of Canada, available at http://www.ncpa.org/sub/dpd/index.php?page=article&Article_ ID=14296 as of August 10, 2009.

17   http://www.sasksurgery.ca/tables/orthopaedic/orthopaedic.htm

18   Hannah Davies, Brisbane Sunday Mail, March 18, 2007, as cited in the Socialized Medicine blog, March 22, 2007, downloaded from http://socglory.blogspot.com/2007/03/nhs-may-be-restricted-to-core-services.html on August 10, 2009.

19   "How Good is Canadian Health Care?," Fraser Institute, December 2006, page 65

20   "B.C. Hospital's Bed Crunch Getting Worse," CBC News, January 30, 2007, downloaded from http://www.cbc.ca/ canada/british-columbia/story/2007/01/30/bc-hospital.html on August 10, 2009.

21   "Back Patients Waiting Years for Treatment: Study," CTV.ca, February 24, 2007, downloaded from http://www. ctv.ca/servlet/ArticleNews/story/CTVNews/20070223/back_patients_070224/20070224?hub=TopStories on August 10, 2009.

22   "How Good is Canadian Health Care?," Fraser Institute, December 2006, page 65

23   Gerald F. Anderson and Peter S. Hussey, "Multinational Comparisons for Health Systems Data," Commonwealth

Fund, October 2000, as cited by John C. Goodman, Gerald L. Musgrave and Devon M. Herrick in "Lives at Risk: Single-Payer National Health Insurance Around the World," Rowan & Littlefield Publishers/National Center for Policy Analysis, 2004, page 73.

24   Gerald F. Anderson and Peter S. Hussey, "Multinational Comparisons for Health Systems Data," Commonwealth Fund, October 2000, as cited by John C. Goodman, Gerald L. Musgrave and Devon M. Herrick in "Lives at Risk: Single-Payer National Health Insurance Around the World," Rowan & Littlefield Publishers/National Center for Policy Analysis, 2004, page 73.

25   Di Caelers, "Surgeon Reveals 18-Year Waiting List for Patients," Cape Argus, March 1, 2007, downloaded from http://www.capeargus.co.za/index.php?fArticleId=3708312 on August 10, 2009.

GREAT BRITAIN

1   "Cataract Surgery," Health Encyclopedia online, National Health Service, available at http://www.nhsdirect.nhs.uk/articles/article.aspx?articleId=89&PrintPage=1 as of July 14, 2009.

2   David Doyle, "Hope in Sight for Richard," Ealing Times (UK), May 29, 2007, available at http://www.ealingtimes.co.uk/mostpopular.var.1432502.mostcommented.hope_in_sight_for_richard.php as of July 14, 2009.

3   Ibid.

4   Ibid.

5   Ibid.

6   Ibid.

7   David Doyle, "Nearly Blind after Three Years' Wait for Eye Op," This Is Local London (UK), May 11, 2007, available at http://www.thisislocallondon.co.uk/mostpopular.var.1391015.mostviewed.nearly_blind_after_three_years_wait_for_eye_op.php as of July 14, 2009.

8   David Doyle, "'He Was a Real English Gentleman,'" Ealing Times (UK), June 27, 2007, available at http://www.thisislocallondon.co.uk/search/1503134._He_was_a_real_English_gentleman_/ as of July 7, 2009.

9   Ibid.

10   Ibid.

11   "Cancer Surgery Postponed Four Times," BBC (UK), January 11, 2000, available at http://newsvote.bbc.co.uk/1/hi/health/598555.stm as of July 7, 2009; Trudy Harris, "Flu Crisis Leads to Critical Delay in Cancer Case," Times (UK), January 14, 2000.

12   Dr. Rebecca Fitzgerald, "Oesophageal Cancer: From Bench to Bedside," University of Cambridge, Cambridge, UK, class lecture, October 4, 2002, available at http://www.cam.ac.uk/cambforall/scienceseminars/cancer/oesophageal.html as of July 7, 2009.

13   "Cancer Inoperable after Flu Delay," BBC (UK), January 13, 2000, available at http://news.bbc.co.uk/1/hi/health/602393.stm as of July 7, 2009.

14   "Cancer Surgery Postponed Four Times," BBC (UK), January 11, 2000, available at http://newsvote.bbc.co.uk/1/hi/health/598555.stm as of July 7, 2009.

15   Stuart Qualtrough, "NHS in Crisis: Destined to Die, a Woman Who Had Faith in the System," Sunday Mirror (UK), January 16, 2000, available at http://findarticles.com/p/articles/mi_qn4161/is_20000116/ai_n9705929/?tag=content;col1 as of July 7, 2009.

16   "Cancer Surgery Postponed Four Times," BBC (UK), January 11, 2000, available at http://newsvote.bbc.co.uk/1/hi/health/598555.stm as of July 7, 2009; Sarah Lyall, "In Britain's Health Service, Sick Itself, Cancer Care Is Dismal," New York Times, February 10, 2000, p. A1, available at http://query.nytimes.com/gst/fullpage.html?sec=health&res=9501EFD9133EF933A25751C0A9669C8B63 as of July 15, 2009.

17   "Cancer Inoperable after Flu Delay," BBC (UK), January 13, 2000, available at http://news.bbc.co.uk/1/hi/health/602393.stm as of July 7, 2009; "Cancer Surgery Postponed Four Times," BBC (UK), January 11, 2000, available at http://newsvote.bbc.co.uk/1/hi/health/598555.stm as of July 7, 2009.

18   "Cancer Surgery Postponed Four Times," BBC (UK), January 11, 2000, available at http://newsvote.bbc.co.uk/1/hi/health/598555.stm as of July 7, 2009.

19   Ibid.

20   Jill Palmer, "Too Busy for Seriously Ill Baby," Mirror (UK), January 11, 2000, p. 2.

21   "Cancer Surgery Postponed Four Times," BBC (UK), January 11, 2000, available at http://newsvote.bbc.co.uk/1/hi/health/598555.stm as of July 7, 2009.

22   Stuart Qualtrough, "NHS in Crisis: Destined to Die, a Woman Who Had Faith in the System," Sunday Mirror (UK), January 16, 2000, available at http://findarticles.com/p/articles/mi_qn4161/is_20000116/ai_n9705929/?tag=content;col1 as of July 7, 2009.

23   Jeremy Laurance, "How Cancelled Operation Highlights Critical Care Bed Bottleneck," Independent (UK), March 4, 2005, p. 4; Kamal Ahmed and Gaby Hinsliff, "Labour's Secret Plans to Storm the NHS Barricades," Observer (UK), April 21, 2002, p. 16; "Cancer Surgery Postponed Four Times," BBC (UK), January 11, 2000, available at http://newsvote.bbc.co.uk/1/hi/health/598555.stm as of July 7, 2009; Trudy Harris, "Flu Crisis Leads to Critical Delay in Cancer Case," Times (UK), January 14, 2000.

24   Trudy Harris, "Flu Crisis Leads to Critical Delay in Cancer Case," Times (UK), January 14, 2000.

25   "Cancer Inoperable after Flu Delay," BBC (UK), January 13, 2000, available at http://news.bbc.co.uk/1/hi/health/602393.stm as of July 7, 2009.

26   Lois Rogers and Michael Prescott, "Knives Out over the NHS Reforms," Sunday Times (UK), June 4, 2000.

27   "Cancer Surgery Postponed Four Times," BBC (UK), January 11, 2000, available at http://newsvote.bbc.co.uk/1/hi/health/598555.stm as of July 7, 2009.

28   Stuart Qualtrough, "NHS in Crisis: Destined to Die, a Woman Who Had Faith in the System," Sunday Mirror (UK), January 16, 2000, available at http://findarticles.com/p/articles/mi_qn4161/is_20000116/ai_n9705929/?tag=content;col1 as of July 7, 2009.

29   Jenny Hope, "Ex-Labour MP Sues NHS for Drug to Save Her Sight," Daily Mail (UK), January 30, 2007.

30   Alice Mahon, "Let Down by NHS in My Fight for Sight," Yorkshire Post (UK), February 15, 2007.

31   "Making Britain Better," Special Report: The NHS at 50, BBC News (UK), August 14, 1998, available at http://news.bbc.co.uk/2/hi/events/nhs_at_50/special_report/119803.stm as of July 7, 2009.

32   See "Macular Degeneration," Health Encyclopedia online, National Health Service, June 27, 2007, available at http://www.nhsdirect.nhs.uk/articles/article.aspx?articleId=399&sectionId=10&PrintPage=1 as of July 7, 2009.

33   Alice Mahon, "Let Down by NHS in My Fight for Sight," Yorkshire Post (UK), February 15, 2007; Jenny Hope, "Ex-Labour MP Sues NHS for Drug to Save Her Sight," Daily Mail (UK), January 30, 2007.

34   Jenny Hope, "Ex-Labour MP Sues NHS for Drug to Save Her Sight," Daily Mail (UK), January 30, 2007.

35   Alice Mahon, "Let Down by NHS in My Fight for Sight," Yorkshire Post (UK), February 15, 2007; Ibid.

36   Jenny Hope, "Ex-Labour MP Sues NHS for Drug to Save Her Sight," Daily Mail (UK), January 30, 2007.

37   Alice Mahon, "To the NHS, Anyone Over 60 is Invisible," Daily Mail (UK), February 13, 2007.

38   Alice Mahon, "Let Down by NHS in My Fight for Sight," Yorkshire Post (UK), February 15, 2007.

39   "PCT Faces Court Battle as Ex-MP Demands Blindness Drug," Sentinel (UK), January 31, 2007.

40   Alice Mahon, "To the NHS, Anyone Over 60 is Invisible," Daily Mail (UK), February 13, 2007.

41   "Threat of Court as Ex-MP Battles to Save Sight," Yorkshire Post (UK), January 30, 2007.

42   Jenny Hope, "Ex-Labour MP Sues NHS for Drug to Save Her Sight," Daily Mail (UK), January 30, 2007.

43   "Former MP Slams U-Turn on Eye Drug Treatment," Yorkshire Post (UK), May 2, 2007.

44   David Derbyshire, "Blindness Drug U-Turn," Daily Mail (UK), August 27, 2008.

45   Beezy Marsh and Georgia Williams, "Patients 'Dying of Dogma,'" Daily Mail (UK), July 27, 2001; Beezy Marsh and Gaby Hinsliff, "NHS Crisis? Blame the Media Says Blair," Daily Mail (UK), March 1, 2000; "Patient Who Got Date a Year after He Died," Express, March 1, 2000.

46   "Surgery a Year Too Late," BBC News (UK), March 1, 2000, available at http://news.bbc.co.uk/2/hi/health/662651.stm as of July 7, 2009.

47   Ibid; Beezy Marsh and Georgia Williams, "Patients 'Dying of Dogma,'" Daily Mail (UK), July 27, 2001.

48   Beezy Marsh and Gaby Hinsliff, "NHS Crisis? Blame the Media Says Blair," Daily Mail (UK), March 1, 2000.

49   Lisa Pritchard, "Op Offer Comes a Year Too Late for Tragic Brian," Western Daily Press (UK), March 1, 2000.

50   "Surgery a Year Too Late," BBC News (UK), March 1, 2000, available at http://news.bbc.co.uk/2/hi/health/662651.stm as of July 7, 2009.

51   Ibid.

52   Chris Maguire, "It's Just Frightening," Bristol Evening Post (UK), April 19, 2001.

53   Lisa Pritchard, "Op Offer Comes a Year Too Late for Tragic Brian," Western Daily Press (UK), March 1, 2000.

54   "The Man Who Turned DIY Dentist," Daily Mail (UK), September 28, 2004.

55   Alastair Taylor, "D.I.Y. Dentist," The Sun (UK), September 28, 2004.

56   "'I Took My Teeth out with Pliers,'" BBC News (UK), September 28, 2007, available at http://news.bbc.co.uk/2/hi/health/3696758.stm as of July 7, 2009.

57   Ibid.

58   Alastair Taylor, "D.I.Y. Dentist," The Sun (UK), September 28, 2004; "'I Took My Teeth out with Pliers,'" BBC News (UK), September 28, 2007, available at http://news.bbc.co.uk/2/hi/health/3696758.stm as of July 7, 2009.

59   "The Man Who Turned DIY Dentist," Daily Mail (UK), September 28, 2004.

60   Alastair Taylor, "D.I.Y. Dentist," The Sun (UK), September 28, 2004.

61   Ibid.

62   "I Yanked My Own Teeth Out," Daily Record (UK), September 28, 2004.

63   "The Man Who Turned DIY Dentist," Daily Mail (UK), September 28, 2004.

64   "George Gets Teeth into New Dentist," Scarborough Evening News (UK), September 29, 2004.

65   "The Man Who Turned DIY Dentist," Daily Mail (UK), September 28, 2004.

66   See "'I Took My Teeth out with Pliers,'" BBC News (UK), September 28, 2007, available at http://news.bbc.co.uk/2/hi/health/3696758.stm as of July 7, 2009.

67   Roland Batten, "New Case of Fighting to Save Sight," This is Wiltshire (UK), June 5, 2007.

68   Ibid.

69   "NHS Leaves Employee to Go Blind," Press Centre, Royal National Institute of Blind People, London, UK, May 18, 2007, available at http://www.rnib.org.uk/xpedio/groups/public/documents/publicwebsite/public_pr180507.hcsp as of July 7, 2009.

70   Ibid.

71   Chris Hooper, "Local Widow Denied Sight-Saving Treatment," This Is Wiltshire (UK), May 26, 2007.

72   Chris Hooper, "Sylvie Wins Fight for Treatment," Salisbury Journal (UK), January 19, 2008, available at http://www.salisburyjournal.co.uk/search/1977820.Sylvie_wins_fight_for_treatment/ as of April 28, 2009.

73   "Threat of Court as Ex-MP Battles to Save Sight," Yorkshire Post (UK), January 30, 2007.

74   "NHS Worker Refused Sight-Saving Drugs," Birmingham Post (UK), May 18, 2007.

75   "Patients Fighting for Blindness Drugs," Press Association Newsfile, June 14, 2007; Roland Batten, "New Case of Fighting to Save Sight," This is Wiltshire (UK), June 5, 2007.

76   "NHS Leaves Employee to Go Blind," Press Centre, Royal National Institute of Blind People, London, UK, May 18, 2007, available at http://www.rnib.org.uk/xpedio/groups/public/documents/publicwebsite/public_pr180507.hcsp as of July 7, 2009.

77   Ibid.

78   Ibid.

79   Ibid.

80   David Derbyshire, "Blindness Drug U-Turn," Daily Mail (UK), August 27, 2008.

81   Chris Hooper, "Sylvie Wins Fight for Treatment," Salisbury Journal (UK), January 19, 2008, available at http://www.salisburyjournal.co.uk/search/1977820.Sylvie_wins_fight_for_treatment/ as of April 28, 2009.

82   Sarah Boseley, "'My Doctor Did Not Tell Me of Life-Saving Drug,'" Guardian (UK), January 5, 2000.

83   Ibid.

84   Ibid.

85   Sarah Lyall, "In Britain's Health Service, Sick Itself, Cancer Care Is Dismal," New York Times, February 10, 2000, available at http://query.nytimes.com/gst/fullpage.html?sec=health&res=9501EFD9133EF933A25751C0A9669C8B63 as of July 7, 2009; Beezy Marsh and Jane Elliott, "Your Money or Your Life," Daily Mail (UK), November 15, 1999.

86   Beezy Marsh and Jane Elliott, "Your Money or Your Life," Daily Mail (UK), November 15, 1999.

87   Sarah Boseley, "'My Doctor Did Not Tell Me of Life-Saving Drug,'" Guardian (UK), January 5, 2000.

88   Sarah Lyall, "In Britain's Health Service, Sick Itself, Cancer Care Is Dismal," New York Times, February 10, 2000, available at http://query.nytimes.com/gst/fullpage.html?sec=health&res=9501EFD9133EF933A25751C0A9669C8B63 as of August 2, 2007.

89   Sarah Boseley, "'My Doctor Did Not Tell Me of Life-Saving Drug,'" Guardian (UK), January 5, 2000.

90   Beezy Marsh and Jane Elliott, "Your Money or Your Life," Daily Mail (UK), November 15, 1999; Ibid.

91   Beezy Marsh and Jane Elliott, "Your Money or Your Life," Daily Mail (UK), November 15, 1999.

92   Ibid.

93   Anjali Kwatra, "Cancer 'Postcode Lottery' Ends," Birmingham Post (UK), April 12, 2000.

94   Sarah Boseley, "'My Doctor Did Not Tell Me of Life-Saving Drug,'" Guardian (UK), January 5, 2000.

95   Beezy Marsh and Jane Elliott, "Doctors 'Have to Beg.'" Daily Mail (UK), November 15, 1999.

96   Beezy Marsh and Jane Elliott, "Your Money or Your Life," Daily Mail (UK), November 15, 1999.

97   Sarah Boseley, "'My Doctor Did Not Tell Me of Life-Saving Drug,'" Guardian (UK), January 5, 2000.

98   Ibid.

99   Beezy Marsh and Jane Elliott, "Your Money or Your Life," Daily Mail (UK), November 15, 1999.

100   Anjali Kwatra, "Cancer 'Postcode Lottery' Ends," Birmingham Post (UK), April 12, 2000.

101   Barbara Argument, "Same Killer, Different Battle," Evening Gazette (UK), February 2, 2005.

102   Steve Doughty and Nick McDermott, "The Woman of 108 Told to Wait 18 Months for Hearing Aid," Daily Mail (UK), available at http://www.dailymail.co.uk/pages/live/articles/news/news.html?in_article_id=471617&in_page_id=1770 as of July 7, 2009; Thair Shaikh, "Woman, 108, Must Wait 18 Months for Hearing Aid," Guardian (UK), July 30, 2007, available at http://www.guardian.co.uk/uk_news/story/0,,2137719,00.html as of July 7, 2009.

103   Steve Doughty and Nick McDermott, "The Woman of 108 Told to Wait 18 Months for Hearing Aid," Daily Mail (UK), available at http://www.dailymail.co.uk/pages/live/articles/news/news.html?in_article_id=471617&in_page_id=1770 as of July 7, 2009.

104   Thair Shaikh, "Woman, 108, Must Wait 18 Months for Hearing Aid," Guardian (UK), July 30, 2007, available at http://www.guardian.co.uk/uk_news/story/0,,2137719,00.html as of July 7, 2009.

105   Steve Doughty and Nick McDermott, "The Woman of 108 Told to Wait 18 Months for Hearing Aid," Daily Mail (UK), available at http://www.dailymail.co.uk/pages/live/articles/news/news.html?in_article_id=471617&in_page_id=1770 as of July 7, 2009.

106   Ibid.

107   Thair Shaikh, "Woman, 108, Must Wait 18 Months for Hearing Aid," Guardian (UK), July 30, 2007, available at http://www.guardian.co.uk/uk_news/story/0,,2137719,00.html as of July 7, 2009.

108   Steve Doughty and Nick McDermott, "The Woman of 108 Told to Wait 18 Months for Hearing Aid," Daily Mail (UK), available at http://www.dailymail.co.uk/pages/live/articles/news/news.html?in_article_id=471617&in_page_id=1770 as of August 7, 2007.

109   Stewart Maclean, "Olive, 108 Gets a Gift of Hearing," Mirror (UK), August 3, 2007, available at http://www.mirror.co.uk/news/topstories/2007/08/03/olive-108-gets-a-gift-of-hearing-89520-19563765/ as of August 7, 2007.

110   Thair Shaikh, "Woman, 108, Must Wait 18 Months for Hearing Aid," Guardian (UK), July 30, 2007, available at http://www.guardian.co.uk/uk_news/story/0,,2137719,00.html as of August 7, 2007.

111   Steve Doughty and Nick McDermott, "The Woman of 108 Told to Wait 18 Months for Hearing Aid," Daily Mail (UK), available at http://www.dailymail.co.uk/pages/live/articles/news/news.html?in_article_id=471617&in_page_id=1770 as of August 7, 2007.

112   Ibid.

113   Ibid.

114   Thair Shaikh, "Woman, 108, Must Wait 18 Months for Hearing Aid," Guardian (UK), July 30, 2007, available at http://www.guardian.co.uk/uk_news/story/0,,2137719,00.html as of August 7, 2007.

115   "Six-Year-Old Dies after Doctors Fail to Diagnose Brain Tumour Eight Times," This Is London (UK), September 8, 2006, available at http://www.thisislondon.co.uk/news/article-23366257-details/Six-year-old+dies+after+doctors+fail+to+diagnose+brain+tumour+eight+times/article.do as of July 7, 2009.

116   Ibid.

117   Ibid; Chris Brooke, "Killed by Tumour, Boy Doctors Sent Home Eight Times," Daily Mail (UK), September 9, 2006.

118   "Six-Year-Old Dies after Doctors Fail to Diagnose Brain Tumour Eight Times," This Is London (UK), September 8, 2006, available at http://www.thisislondon.co.uk/news/article-23366257-details/Six-year-old+dies+after+doctors+fail+to+diagnose+brain+tumour+eight+times/article.do as of July 7, 2009.

119   Chris Brooke, "Killed by Tumour, Boy Doctors Sent Home Eight Times," Daily Mail (UK), September 9, 2006.

120   Mark Lavery, "Brain Tumour Boy's Mum Attacks Doctors," Yorkshire Evening Post (UK), September 9, 2006, available at http://www.yorkshireeveningpost.co.uk/ViewArticle.aspx?SectionID=39&ArticleID=1757248 as of July 7, 2009.

121   "Six-Year-Old Dies after Doctors Fail to Diagnose Brain Tumour Eight Times," This Is London (UK), September 8, 2006, available at http://www.thisislondon.co.uk/news/article-23366257-details/Six-year-old+dies+after+doctors+fail+to+diagnose+brain+tumour+eight+times/article.do as of July 7, 2009.

122   Alistair Keely, "Hospital Bosses to Meet Tumour Tragedy Row Mother," Press Association Newsfile, September 8, 2006.

123   Mark Lavery, "Brain Tumour Boy's Mum Attacks Doctors," Yorkshire Evening Post (UK), September 9, 2006, available at http://www.yorkshireeveningpost.co.uk/ViewArticle.aspx?SectionID=39&ArticleID=1757248 as of July 7, 2009.

124   "Six-Year-Old Dies after Doctors Fail to Diagnose Brain Tumour Eight Times," This Is London (UK), September 8, 2006, available at http://www.thisislondon.co.uk/news/article-23366257-details/Six-year-old+dies+after+doctors+fail+to+diagnose+brain+tumour+eight+times/article.do as of July 7, 2009.

125   Ibid.

126   Ibid.

127   Mark Lavery, "Brain Tumour Boy's Mum Attacks Doctors," Yorkshire Evening Post (UK), September 9, 2006, available at http://www.yorkshireeveningpost.co.uk/ViewArticle.aspx?SectionID=39&ArticleID=1757248 as of July 7, 2009.

128   Chris Brooke, "Killed by Tumour, Boy Doctors Sent Home Eight Times," Daily Mail (UK), September 9, 2006.

129   Mark Lavery, "Brain Tumour Boy's Mum Attacks Doctors," Yorkshire Evening Post (UK), September 9, 2006, available at http://www.yorkshireeveningpost.co.uk/ViewArticle.aspx?SectionID=39&ArticleID=1757248 as of July 7, 2009.

130   "Six-Year-Old Dies after Doctors Fail to Diagnose Brain Tumour Eight Times," This Is London (UK), September 8, 2006, available at http://www.thisislondon.co.uk/news/article-23366257-details/Six-year-old+dies+after+doctors+fail+to+diagnose+brain+tumour+eight+times/article.do as of July 7, 2009.

131   "Family Fights for Justice," Wakefield Express (UK), March 6, 2007, available at http://www.wakefieldexpress.co.uk/ViewArticle.aspx?SectionID=702&articleid=2100303 as of August 21, 2007.

132   Lindsay Pantry, "'Serious' Errors Investigated at Hospital Trust," Wakefield Express (UK), April 30, 2009, available at http://www.wakefieldexpress.co.uk/news/39Serious39-errors-investigated-at-hospital.5201086.jp as of May 1, 2009.

133   Ibid.

134   Betty Anderson, "Finn, 5, Waits in Agony for Dentist," Wilmslow Express (UK), March 29, 2006, available at http://www.thewilmslowexpress.co.uk/news/s/211/211087_finn_5_waits_in_agony_for_dentist.html as of July 7, 2009; Paul Broster, "Labour Claims It is Boosting NHS Dentists," Express (UK), March 31, 2006.

135   Bill Martin, "Throbsmacked," Daily Star (UK), March 31, 2006.

136   Betty Anderson, "Finn, 5, Waits in Agony for Dentist," Wilmslow Express (UK), March 29, 2006, available at http://www.thewilmslowexpress.co.uk/news/s/211/211087_finn_5_waits_in_agony_for_dentist.html as of July 7, 2009.

137   Ibid.

138   Bill Martin, "Throbsmacked," Daily Star (UK), March 31, 2006.

139   Betty Anderson, "Finn, 5, Waits in Agony for Dentist," Wilmslow Express (UK), March 29, 2006, available at http://www.thewilmslowexpress.co.uk/news/s/211/211087_finn_5_waits_in_agony_for_dentist.html as of July 7, 2009.

140   Ibid.

141   Paul Broster, "Labour Claims It is Boosting NHS Dentists," Express (UK), March 31, 2006.

142   Betty Anderson, "Finn, 5, Waits in Agony for Dentist," Wilmslow Express (UK), March 29, 2006, available at http://www.thewilmslowexpress.co.uk/news/s/211/211087_finn_5_waits_in_agony_for_dentist.html as of July 7, 2009.

143   Paul Broster, "Labour Claims It is Boosting NHS Dentists," Express (UK), March 31, 2006.

144   Betty Anderson, "Finn, 5, Waits in Agony for Dentist," Wilmslow Express (UK), March 29, 2006, available at http://www.thewilmslowexpress.co.uk/news/s/211/211087_finn_5_waits_in_agony_for_dentist.html as of July 7, 2009.

145   Betty Anderson, "Young Toothache Victim Gets Welcome Relief," Manchester Evening News (UK), April 26, 2006, available at http://www.manchestereveningnews.co.uk/news/s/512/512184_young_toothache_victim_gets_welcome_relief.html as of July 7, 2009.

146   Ibid.

147   Andrew Levy, "The Hospital of Horrors," Daily Mail (UK), August 18, 2007; David Sapsted, "NHS Shortages Force Lavatory Birth," Daily Telegraph (UK), August 18, 2007.

148   Andrew Levy, "The Hospital of Horrors," Daily Mail (UK), August 18, 2007; "The Plot Sickens," Investor's Business Daily, August 23, 2007, available at http://www.ibdeditorials.com/IBDArticles.aspx?id=272674493362777 as of July 7, 2009.

149   Andrew Levy, "The Hospital of Horrors," Daily Mail (UK), August 18, 2007; Yepoka Yeebo, "Baby's Birth and Death in Lavatory of Hospital with No Trained Staff," Times (UK), August 18, 2007.

150   David Sapsted, "NHS Shortages Force Lavatory Birth," Daily Telegraph (UK), August 18, 2007; Jo Willey, "Mother Sees Baby Die after Being Left to Give Birth in Hospital Toilet," Express (UK), August 18, 2007.

151   Jo Willey, "Mother Sees Baby Die after Being Left to Give Birth in Hospital Toilet," Express (UK), August 18, 2007.

152   Ibid; "Mum Left to Deliver Dead Son," Mirror (UK), August 18, 2007; Andrew Levy, "The Hospital of Horrors," Daily Mail (UK), August 18, 2007.

153   Jo Willey, "Mother Sees Baby Die after Being Left to Give Birth in Hospital Toilet," Express (UK), August 18, 2007.

154   Ibid.

155   Yepoka Yeebo, "Baby's Birth and Death in Lavatory of Hospital with No Trained Staff," Times (UK), August 18, 2007.

156   Jo Willey, "Mother Sees Baby Die after Being Left to Give Birth in Hospital Toilet," Express (UK), August 18, 2007.

157   Yepoka Yeebo, "Baby's Birth and Death in Lavatory of Hospital with No Trained Staff," Times (UK), August 18, 2007; Andrew Levy, "The Hospital of Horrors," Daily Mail (UK), August 18, 2007.

158   "Mum's Ordeal," Brentwood Gazette (UK), August 22, 2007.

159   Andrew Levy, "The Hospital of Horrors," Daily Mail (UK), August 18, 2007.

160   "Mother's 35-Minute Ambulance Wait," BBC News (UK), August 16, 2007, available at http://news.bbc.co.uk/1/hi/england/devon/6949680.stm as of July 7, 2009.

161   "Baby's 35-Minute Ambulance Wait," This Is Cornwall (UK), August 16, 2007.

162   Ibid.

163   Ibid.

164   Ibid.

165   Ibid.

166   Ibid.

167   "Mother's 35-Minute Ambulance Wait," BBC News (UK), August 16, 2007, available at http://news.bbc.co.uk/1/hi/england/devon/6949680.stm as of July 7, 2009; Ibid.

168   "Baby's 35-Minute Ambulance Wait," This Is Cornwall (UK), August 16, 2007.

169   "Factsheet: Ambulance Trust," Department of Health, South Western Ambulance Service NHS Trust, July 6, 2007; "Baby's 35-Minute Ambulance Wait," This Is Cornwall (UK), August 16, 2007.

170   "Baby's 35-Minute Ambulance Wait," This Is Cornwall (UK), August 16, 2007.

171   Ibid.

172   Chris Brooke, "Mum Gives Birth in Car Park Because 'Hospital Didn't Have Midwife,'" Daily Mail (UK), August 29, 2007, available at http://www.dailymail.co.uk/pages/live/articles/news/news.html?in_article_id=478510&in_page_id=1770 as of July 8, 2009; Robin Perrie, "New Mum's Pain and Display," Sun (UK), August 30, 2007, available at http://www.thesun.co.uk/article/0,,2-2007400341,00.html as of September 10, 2007; "Parents' Fury over Birth in Car Park," Scarborough Evening News (UK), August 31, 2007, available at http://www.scarboroughevening news.co.uk/news/Parents-fury-overbirth-in-car.3163048.jp as of July 8, 2009.

173   Chris Brooke, "Mum Gives Birth in Car Park Because 'Hospital Didn't Have Midwife,'" Daily Mail (UK), August 29, 2007, available at http://www.dailymail.co.uk/pages/live/articles/news/news.html?in_article_id=478510&in_page_id=1770 as of July 8, 2009.

174   Mark Foster, "Car Park Birth Parents Angered by Closure Plans," Northern Echo (UK), August 30, 2007, available at http://www.thenorthernecho.co.uk/news/health/display.var.1652237.0.car_park_birth_parents_angered_by_closure_plans.php as of July 8, 2009.

175   "Hospital Tells Mother to Phone 999," Metro (UK), August 29, 2007, available at http://www.metro.co.uk/news/article.html?in_article_id=63944&in_page_id=34 as of July 8, 2009.

176   Robin Perrie, "New Mum's Pain and Display," Sun (UK), August 30, 2007, available at http://www.thesun.co.uk/article/0,,2-2007400341,00.html as of September 10, 2007.

177   "Parents' Fury over Birth in Car Park," Scarborough Evening News (UK), August 31, 2007, available at http://www.scarborougheveningnews.co.uk/news/Parents-fury-overbirth-in-car.3163048.jp as of July 8, 2009.

178   Chris Brooke, "Mum Gives Birth in Car Park Because 'Hospital Didn't Have Midwife,'" Daily Mail (UK), August 29, 2007, available at http://www.dailymail.co.uk/pages/live/articles/news/news.html?in_article_id=478510&in_page_id=1770 as of July 8, 2009.

179   Ibid.

180   "Baby Born in Hospital's Car Park," BBC (UK), August 30, 2007, available at http://news.bbc.co.uk/1/hi/england/north_yorkshire/6970457.stm as of July 8, 2009.

181   "Cancer Victim's Agony over Refusal of Drug," Cambridge Evening News (UK), April 10, 2006.

182   Severin Carrell, "Cancer: The Postcode Lottery that Saved Brian of SO42 and Doomed James of CB2," Independent (UK), April 9, 2006.

183   Ibid.

184   For example, see Patrick Butler, "Q&A: Postcode Lottery," Guardian (UK), November 9, 2000, available at http://society.guardian.co.uk/nhsperformance/story/0,,395004,00.html as of July 8, 2009.

185   Severin Carrell, "Cancer: The Postcode Lottery that Saved Brian of SO42 and Doomed James of CB2," Independent (UK), April 9, 2006.

186   Harriet Harman, "Trust to Pay for Cancer Drug," Independent (UK), May 14, 2006; "Cancer Victim's Agony over Refusal of Drug," Cambridge Evening News (UK), April 10, 2006.

187   Severin Carrell, "Cancer: The Postcode Lottery that Saved Brian of SO42 and Doomed James of CB2," Independent (UK), April 9, 2006.

188   "Wrong Address: The Pounds 15,000 Price Tag on a Man's Future," Independent (UK), April 9, 2006.

189   "Cancer Victim's Agony over Refusal of Drug," Cambridge Evening News (UK), April 10, 2006.

190   Severin Carrell, "Cancer: The Postcode Lottery that Saved Brian of SO42 and Doomed James of CB2," Independent (UK), April 9, 2006.

191   Harriet Harman, "Trust to Pay for Cancer Drug," Independent (UK), May 14, 2006.

192   Chris Brooke, "Doctors Refuse to Fix Builder's Broken Ankle Unless He Quits Smoking," Daily Mail (UK), September 13, 2007, available at http://www.dailymail.co.uk/pages/live/articles/news/news.html?in_article_id=481617&in_page_id=1770&ct=5 as of July 9, 2009.

193   John Coles, "Smoker Refused Surgery on NHS," Sun (UK), September 14, 2007, available at http://www.thesun.co.uk/article/0,,2-2007420800,00.html as of September 19, 2007.

194   "No Surgery unless You Quit, Smoker Told by Hospital," This Is Cornwall (UK), September 13, 2007, available at http://www.thisiscornwall.co.uk/displayNode.jsp?nodeId=146868&command=displayContent&sourceNode=146861&contentPK=18382251&folderPk=83306&pNodeId=146875 as of September 19, 2007.

195   Ibid.

196   Chris Brooke, "Doctors Refuse to Fix Builder's Broken Ankle Unless He Quits Smoking," Daily Mail (UK), September 13, 2007, available at http://www.dailymail.co.uk/pages/live/articles/news/news.html?in_article_id=481617&in_page_id=1770&ct=5 as of July 9, 2009.

197   "No Surgery Unless You Quit, Smoker Told by Hospital," This Is Cornwall (UK), September 13, 2007, available at http://www.thisiscornwall.co.uk/displayNode.jsp?nodeId=146868&command=displayContent&sourceNode=146861&contentPK=18382251&folderPk=83306&pNodeId=146875 as of September 19, 2007.

198   John Coles, "Smoker Refused Surgery on NHS," Sun (UK), September 14, 2007, available at http://www.thesun.co.uk/article/0,,2-2007420800,00.html as of September 19, 2007.

199   Dan Newling, "Smokers Told to Quit or Surgery Will Be Refused," Daily Mail (UK), June 3, 2007, available at http://www.dailymail.co.uk/pages/live/articles/news/news.html?in_article_id=459574&in_page_id=1770 as of September 19, 2007.

200   John Coles, "Smoker Refused Surgery on NHS," Sun (UK), September 14, 2007, available at http://www.thesun.co.uk/article/0,,2-2007420800,00.html as of September 19, 2007.

201   "Patient Told: No Smoking Pledge, No Operation," Western Morning News (UK), September 14, 2007.

202   John Coles, "Smoker Refused Surgery on NHS," Sun (UK), September 14, 2007, available at http://www.thesun.co.uk/article/0,,2-2007420800,00.html as of September 19, 2007.

203   "Patient Told: No Smoking Pledge, No Operation," Western Morning News (UK), September 14, 2007.

204   Chris Brooke, "Doctors Refuse to Fix Builder's Broken Angle unless He Quits Smoking," Daily Mail (UK), September 13, 2007, available at http://www.dailymail.co.uk/pages/live/articles/news/news.html?in_article_id=481617&in_page_id=1770&ct=5 as of July 9, 2009.

205   "Patient Told: No Smoking Pledge, No Operation," Western Morning News (UK), September 14, 2007.

206   Details for this story were obtained from Emma Morton, "Home-Birth Hell after Ward Snub," Sun (UK), August 31, 2007, available at http://www.thesun.co.uk/article/0,,2-2007400576,00.html as of July 9, 2009, and Siobhan Ryan, "Mum's Terror at Home Birth," Argus (UK), August 31, 2007, available at http://www.theargus.co.uk/misc/print.php?artid=1656981 as of July 9, 2009.

207   For all source material, see Catherine Pye, "Burns Man's DIY Warning," Blackburn, Darwen and Hyndburn Citizen (UK), September 17, 2007, available at http://www.blackburncitizen.co.uk/misc/print.php?artid=1693123 as of July 9, 2009.

208   "Clinical Expectations to the 4 Hour Emergency Care Target," Department of Health, United Kingdom, p. 1, available at http://www.dh.gov.uk/prod_consum_dh/groups/dh_digitalassets/@dh/@en/documents/digitalasset/dh_4079556.pdf as of September 25, 2007.

209   For all source material and references, see Katie Campling, "No Room for Baby Joseph," Huddersfield Daily Examiner (UK), October 1, 2007, available at http://ichuddersfield.icnetwork.co.uk/examiner/news/regional/tm_headline=no-room-for-baby-joseph&method=full&objectid=19875320&siteid=50060-name_page.html as of June 23, 2009.

210   Sarah Boseley, "Patients Pull Own Teeth as Dental Contract Falters," Guardian (UK), October 15, 2007, available at http://www.guardian.co.uk/medicine/story/0,,2191204,00.html as of July 9, 2009.

211   "'I Rip Out My Teeth with Pliers,'" BBC News (UK), October 15, 2007, available at http://news.bbc.co.uk/1/hi/health/7045143.stm as of July 9, 2009.

212   Ibid.

213   Ibid.

214   Ibid.

215   Ibid.

216   Ibid.

217   Sarah Boseley, "Patients Pull Own Teeth as Dental Contract Falters," Guardian (UK), October 15, 2007, available at http://www.guardian.co.uk/medicine/story/0,,2191204,00.html as of July 9, 2009; Jenny Hope, "Patients Turn to DIY Dentistry as the Crisis in NHS Care Deepens," Daily Mail (UK), October 14, 2007, available at http://www.dailymail.co.uk/pages/live/articles/news/news.html?in_article_id=487621&in_page_id=1770&ct=5 as of July 9, 2009; "Brits Resort to Pulling Own Teeth," CNN, October 15, 2007, available at http://www.cnn.com/2007/WORLD/europe/10/15/england.dentists/index.html as of July 9, 2009.

218   Sarah Boseley, "Patients Pull Own Teeth as Dental Contract Falters," Guardian (UK), October 15, 2007, available at http://www.guardian.co.uk/medicine/story/0,,2191204,00.html as of July 9, 2009.

219   John Howard, "Dental Patients 'Removing Own Teeth,'" Suffolk and Essex Online (UK), October 15, 2007, available at http://www.eadt.co.uk/content/eadt/news/story.aspx?brand=EADOnline&category=News&tBrand=EADOnline&tCategory=News&itemid=IPED14%20Oct%202007%2022%3A56%3A18%3A997 as of July 9, 2009.

220   Jo Willey, "The Patients Forced to Pull out Their Own Teeth," Daily Express (UK), October 15, 2007, available at http://www.express.co.uk/posts/view/22071/The-patients-forced-to-pull-out-their-own-teeth as of July 9, 2009.

221   Matthew Parris, "Patients Feel the Pain in NHS Dental Crisis," Times (UK), October 15, 2007, available at http://www.timesonline.co.uk/tol/life_and_style/health/article2659300.ece as of July 9, 2009.

222   "Year-Long Wait for NHS Dentist," Sunderland Echo (UK), October 15, 2007, available at http://www.sunderlandecho.com/news/Yearlong-wait-for-NHS-dentist.3377540.jp as of July 9, 2009; "Patients Overwhelm NHS Dentists," BBC News (UK), November 1, 2006, available at http://news.bbc.co.uk/1/hi/england/cornwall/6105042.stm as of July 9, 2009.

223   "'I Rip out My Teeth with Pliers,'" BBC News (UK), October 15, 2007, available at http://news.bbc.co.uk/1/hi/health/7045143.stm as of July 9, 2009.

224   "Taxi Driver Pulls Own Teeth out with Pliers Due to Long Waiting Lists for NHS Dentists," Daily Mail (UK), October 19, 2007, available at http://www.dailymail.co.uk/pages/live/articles/news/news.html?in_article_id=488569&in_page_id=1770 as of July 9, 2009.

225   Alan Thompson, "The DIY Dentist," Leicester Mercury, October 19, 2007.

226   "Taxi Driver Pulls Own Teeth out with Pliers Due to Long Waiting Lists for NHS Dentists," Daily Mail (UK), October 19, 2007, available at http://www.dailymail.co.uk/pages/live/articles/news/news.html?in_article_id=488569&in_page_id=1770 as of July 9, 2009.

227   "Man Rips out Teeth to Beat Queue," Herald Sun (Australia), October 22, 2007, available at http://www.news.com.au/heraldsun/story/0,21985,22626453-5002700,00.html as of July 9, 2009.

228   "Taxi Driver Pulls Own Teeth out with Pliers Due to Long Waiting Lists for NHS Dentists," Daily Mail (UK), October 19, 2007, available at http://www.dailymail.co.uk/pages/live/articles/news/news.html?in_article_id=488569&in_page_id=1770 as of July 9, 2009.

229   "Man Pulls Own Teeth Out," Press Association (UK), October 20, 2007.

230   "Taxi Driver Pulls Own Teeth out with Pliers Due to Long Waiting Lists for NHS Dentists," Daily Mail (UK), October 19, 2007, available at http://www.dailymail.co.uk/pages/live/articles/news/news.html?in_article_id=488569&in_page_id=1770 as of July 9, 2009.

231   Alan Thompson, "The DIY Dentist," Leicester Mercury, October 19, 2007.

232   Andrew Parker, "DIY Op Cabbie Pulled 6 Teeth," Sun (UK), October 20, 2007, available at http://www.thesun.co.uk/sol/homepage/news/article366040.ece as of July 9, 2009.

233   Alan Thompson, "The DIY Dentist," Leicester Mercury, October 19, 2007.

234   Ibid.

235   Stephen Ellis, "Know the Drill for Non-NHS Tooth Care," Telegraph (UK), October 20, 2007, available at http://www.telegraph.co.uk/money/main.jhtml?xml=/money/2007/10/19/cmdentist20.xml&DCMP=ILC-traffdrv07053100 as of July 9, 2009; "Taxi Driver Pulls Own Teeth out with Pliers Due to Long Waiting Lists for NHS Dentists," Daily Mail (UK), October 19, 2007, available at http://www.dailymail.co.uk/pages/live/articles/news/news.html?in_article_id=488569&in_page_id=1770 as of October 23, 2007.

236   "Taxi Driver Pulls Own Teeth out with Pliers Due to Long Waiting Lists for NHS Dentists," Daily Mail (UK), October 19, 2007, available at http://www.dailymail.co.uk/pages/live/articles/news/news.html?in_article_id=488569&in_page_id=1770 as of July 9, 2009.

237   Stephen Ellis, "Know the Drill for Non-NHS Tooth Care," Telegraph (UK), October 20, 2007, available at http://www.telegraph.co.uk/money/main.jhtml?xml=/money/2007/10/19/cmdentist20.xml&DCMP=ILC-traffdrv07053100 as of July 9, 2009.

238   "Taxi Driver Pulls Own Teeth out with Pliers Due to Long Waiting Lists for NHS Dentists," Daily Mail (UK), October 19, 2007, available at http://www.dailymail.co.uk/pages/live/articles/news/news.html?in_article_id=488569&in_page_id=1770 as of July 9, 2009.

239   Pat Hagan, "I Yanked Tooth Out with My Nails," Sun (UK), October 16, 2007, available at http://www.thesun.co.uk/sol/homepage/news/article345741.ece as of July 9, 2009; "'I Was Left to Pull Out My Own Tooth,'" Prestwich Advertiser (UK), October 18, 2007, available at http://www.prestwichadvertiser.co.uk/news/s/533439_i_was_left_to_pull_out_my_own_tooth as of October 26, 2007.

240   "'I Was Left to Pull Out My Own Tooth,'" Prestwich Advertiser (UK), October 18, 2007, available at http://www.prestwichadvertiser.co.uk/news/s/533439_i_was_left_to_pull_out_my_own_tooth as of July 9, 2009.

241   Pat Hagan, "I Yanked Tooth Out with My Nails," Sun (UK), October 16, 2007, available at http://www.thesun.co.uk/sol/homepage/news/article345741.ece as of July 9, 2009; Ibid.

242   Pat Hagan, "I Yanked Tooth Out with My Nails," Sun (UK), October 16, 2007, available at http://www.thesun.co.uk/sol/homepage/news/article345741.ece as of July 9, 2009; "'I Was Left to Pull Out My Own Tooth,'" Prestwich Advertiser (UK), October 18, 2007, available at http://www.prestwichadvertiser.co.uk/news/s/533439_i_was_left_to_pull_out_my_own_tooth as of July 9, 2009.

243   Pat Hagan, "I Yanked Tooth Out with My Nails," Sun (UK), October 16, 2007, available at http://www.thesun.co.uk/sol/homepage/news/article345741.ece as of July 9, 2009.

244   "'I Was Left to Pull Out My Own Tooth,'" Prestwich Advertiser (UK), October 18, 2007, available at http://www.prestwichadvertiser.co.uk/news/s/533439_i_was_left_to_pull_out_my_own_tooth as of July 9, 2009.

245   Ibid; Pat Hagan, "I Yanked Tooth Out with My Nails," Sun (UK), October 16, 2007, available at http://www.thesun.co.uk/sol/homepage/news/article345741.ece as of July 9, 2009.

246   Pat Hagan, "I Yanked Tooth Out with My Nails," Sun (UK), October 16, 2007, available at http://www.thesun.co.uk/sol/homepage/news/article345741.ece as of October 26, 2007.

247   Amanda Crook, "Woman Extracts Own Tooth," Manchester Evening News (UK), October 16, 2007, available at http://www.manchestereveningnews.co.uk/news/health/s/1019983_woman_extracts_own_tooth as of July 9, 2009.

248   "'I Was Left to Pull Out My Own Tooth,'" Prestwich Advertiser (UK), October 18, 2007, available at http://www.prestwichadvertiser.co.uk/news/s/533439_i_was_left_to_pull_out_my_own_tooth as of July 9, 2009.

249   Sue Carroll, "Driven to Extraction by a Dental Disaster," Mirror (UK), October 17, 2007, available at http://www.mirror.co.uk/news/columnists/carroll/2007/10/17/driven-to-extraction-by-a-dental-disaster-89520-19963629/ as of July 9, 2009.

250   "Dental Patients Face 40-Mile Trip," BBC News (UK), March 22, 2006, available at http://news.bbc.co.uk/2/hi/uk_news/england/cornwall/4831718.stm as of July 9, 2009.

251   "Specialist Dentistry Work to Be Limited," Scunthorpe Telegraph (UK), October 20, 2007.

252   Amy Iggulden, "NHS Dentists Turn Away Patients with Bad Teeth," Telegraph (UK), May 28, 2007, available at http://www.telegraph.co.uk/news/main.jhtml?xml=/news/2007/05/28/nhs28.xml as of July 9, 2009.

253   For all source material and references, unless otherwise noted, see Patrick Sawer and Laura Donnelly, "British Health Case Studies," Sunday Telegraph (UK), October 28, 2007, available at http://www.telegraph.co.uk/news/main.jhtml?xml=/news/2007/10/28/nhealth628.xml as of July 9, 2009.

254   Martin McKeown, "More Tourists Opt for a New Face in the Sun," Express (UK), April 13, 2008.

255   Laura Donnelly and Patrick Sawer, "Record Numbers Go Abroad for Health," Sunday Telegraph (UK), October 28, 2007, available at http://www.telegraph.co.uk/news/main.jhtml?xml=/news/2007/10/28/nhealth128.xml as of July 9, 2009.

256   "Tourism Can Be Healthy Option," Express (UK), October 2, 2008.

257   For all source material and references, see Isla Whitcroft, "Killed by a Hospital that Just Didn't Care – A Widow Recounts her Husband's Final Days," Daily Mail (UK), October 31, 2007, available at http://www.dailymail.co.uk/pages/live/articles/health/healthmain.html?in_article_id=490583&in_page_id=1774&ct=5 as of June 23, 2009.

258   For all source material and references, unless otherwise noted, see "Pensioner Spends Life Savings on Vital Op after NHS Cancels Four Times," Daily Mail (UK), November 2, 2007, available at http://www.dailymail.co.uk/pages/live/articles/health/healthmain.html?in_article_id=491275 as of July 9, 2009.

259   "Still Waiting at Hospitals?," Channel 4 News (UK), June 1, 2007, available at http://www.channel4.com/news/articles/politics/domestic_politics/still+waiting+at+hospitals/978877 as of July 9, 2009.

260   Unless otherwise specified, the source for this story is Mary McConnell, "Hospital Transport Unit Condemned by Patient," The Press (UK), September 7, 2007 and Tan Parsons, "Three Hours for a 12-Minute Journey? This is Madness," Hampstead and Highgate Express (UK), September 13, 2007.

261   Nottingham University report cited from "Four-Hour Wait for Dialysis Treatment," Nottingham Evening Post (UK), November 9, 2007.

262   Alison Smith-Squire, "My Father Was Treated Worse than an Animal in Hospital," Daily Mail (UK), November 6, 2007, available at http://www.dailymail.co.uk/pages/live/articles/health/healthmain.html?in_article_id=491984&in_page_id=1774&in_a_source as of July 9, 2009; "We Treat Horses Better than the NHS Treated My Father, Says Jenny Pitman," Daily Mail (UK), October 23, 2007, available at http://www.dailymail.co.uk/pages/live/articles/news/news.html?in_article_id=489314&in_page_id=1770&ito=1490 as of November 21, 2007.

263   Barry Leightonb, "Hospital Denies Giving Retired Farmer a Killer Superbug," Western Daily Press (UK), October 26, 2007.

264   Alison Smith-Squire, "My Father Was Treated Worse Than an Animal in Hospital," Daily Mail (UK), November 6, 2007, available at http://www.dailymail.co.uk/pages/live/articles/health/healthmain.html?in_article_id=491984&in_page_id=1774&in_a_source as of July 9, 2009.

265   Ibid.

266   Ibid.

267   For instance, see "Superbug Hospital Will Not Be Prosecuted," Reuters, November 15, 2007, available at http://uk.reuters.com/article/domesticNews/idUKL1544257220071115 as of July 9, 2009; Victoria Fletcher, "How Hospital Bug Killed 90 Patients," Daily Express (UK), October 11, 2007, available at http://www.express.co.uk/posts/view/21674/How-hospital-bug-killed-90-patients as of July 9, 2009; Lyndsay Moss, "Deaths from Superbug Soaring," Scotsman (UK), October 24, 2007.

268   Polly Curtis and John Carvel, "Deaths Caused by Two Superbugs Soar as Health Inspectorate Accuses Government," Guardian (UK), February 23, 2007, available at http://www.guardiàn.co.uk/uk_news/story/0,,2019317,00.html as of July 9, 2009.

269   Alison Smith-Squire, "My Father Was Treated Worse than an Animal in Hospital," Daily Mail (UK), November 6, 2007, available at http://www.dailymail.co.uk/pages/live/articles/health/healthmain.html?in_article_id=491984&in_page_id=1774&in_a_source as of July 9, 2009.

270   Ibid.

271   Ibid.

272   Ibid.

273   Ibid.

274   "Horse Trainer Tells of Father's Death," Swindon Advertiser (UK), October 25, 2007, available at http://www.swindonadvertiser.co.uk/news/swindonnewsheadlines/display.var.1785319.0.horse_trainer_tells_of_fathers_death.php as of July 9, 2009.

275   Alison Smith-Squire, "My Father Was Treated Worse than an Animal in Hospital," Daily Mail (UK), November 6, 2007, available at http://www.dailymail.co.uk/pages/live/articles/health/healthmain.html?in_article_id=491984&in_page_id=1774&in_a_source as of July9, 2009.

276   "We Treat Horses Better than the NHS Treated My Father, Says Jenny Pitman," Daily Mail (UK), October 23, 2007, available at http://www.dailymail.co.uk/pages/live/articles/news/news.html?in_article_id=489314&in_page_id=1770&ito=1490 as of July 15, 2009.

277   "Horse Trainer Tells of Father's Death," Swindon Advertiser (UK), October 25, 2007, available at http://www.swindonadvertiser.co.uk/news/swindonnewsheadlines/display.var.1785319.0.horse_trainer_tells_of_fathers_death.php as of July 9, 2009.

278   "We Treat Horses Better than the NHS Treated My Father, Says Jenny Pitman," Daily Mail (UK), October 23, 2007, available at http://www.dailymail.co.uk/pages/live/articles/news/news.html?in_article_id=489314&in_page_id=1770&ito=1490 as of July 15, 2009.

279   Alison Smith-Squire, "My Father Was Treated Worse than an Animal in Hospital," Daily Mail (UK), November 6, 2007, available at http://www.dailymail.co.uk/pages/live/articles/health/healthmain.html?in_article_id=491984&in_page_id=1774&in_a_source as of July 9, 2009.

280   See "Horse Trainer Tells of Father's Death," Swindon Advertiser (UK), October 25, 2007, available at http://www.swindonadvertiser.co.uk/news/swindonnewsheadlines/display.var.1785319.0.horse_trainer_tells_of_fathers_death.php as of July 9, 2009.

281   The Care Quality Commission replaced the Healthcare Commission in April 2009.

282   "Investigation into Outbreaks of Clostridium difficile at Maidstone and Tunbridge Wells NHS Trust," Healthcare Commission, October 2007, p. 38, available at http://news.bbc.co.uk/1/shared/bsp/hi/pdfs/11_10_07maidstone_and_tunbridge_wells_investigation_report_oct_2007.pdf as of May 22, 2009.

283   "Year-Long Wait for Pain Relief," Cambridge Evening News (UK), September 7, 2007.

284   Ibid; "Sufferer Slams Hospital 'Delay,'" Newmarket Journal (UK), September 19, 2007, available at http://www.newmarketjournal.co.uk/news/Sufferer-slams-hospital-39delay39.3215579.jp as of November 27, 2007.

285   "Sufferer Slams Hospital 'Delay,'" Newmarket Journal (UK), September 19, 2007, available at http://www.newmarketjournal.co.uk/news/Sufferer-slams-hospital-39delay39.3215579.jp as of July 9, 2009.

286   Ibid.

287   Ibid.

288   "Year-Long Wait for Pain Relief," Cambridge Evening News (UK), September 7, 2007.

289   "Sufferer Slams Hospital 'Delay,'" Newmarket Journal (UK), September 19, 2007, available at http://www.newmarketjournal.co.uk/news/Sufferer-slams-hospital-39delay39.3215579.jp as of July 9, 2009.

290   "Year-Long Wait for Pain Relief," Cambridge Evening News (UK), September 7, 2007.

291   Ibid.

292   Ibid.

293   "I'm a Patient – 18 Weeks Pathway," National Health Service, available at http://www.18weeks.nhs.uk/Content.aspx?path=/What-is-18-weeks/patient as of July 9, 2009.

294   "Year-Long Wait for Pain Relief," Cambridge Evening News (UK), September 7, 2007.

295   "Sufferer Slams Hospital 'Delay,'" Newmarket Journal (UK), September 19, 2007, available at http://www.newmarketjournal.co.uk/news/Sufferer-slams-hospital-39delay39.3215579.jp as of July 9, 2009.

296   Ibid.

297   Unless otherwise noted, for all source material and references, see Rachel Ellis, "Maternity Meltdown," Daily Mail (UK), March 27, 2007, available at http://www.dailymail.co.uk/pages/live/articles/health/womenfamily.html?in_article_id=444833&in_page_id=1774&ito=1490 as of July 9, 2009.

298   The Care Quality Commission replaced the Healthcare Commission in April 2009.

299   "Women's Experiences of Maternity Care in the NHS in England," Healthcare Commission (London, UK), November 2007, p. 5, available at http://www.healthcarecommission.org.uk/_db/_documents/Maternity_services_survey_report.pdf as of November 29, 2007.

300   Janine Maher, "Mums Say NHS Maternity Services are Good in Biggest ever Survey," Healthcare Commission (London, UK), November 27, 2007, available at http://www.healthcarecommission.org.uk/newsandevents/pressreleases.cfm?cit_id=5931&FAArea1=customWidgets.content_view_1&usecache=false as of November 29, 2007.

301   For all references and source material, see Emma Morton, "Docs Missed Cancer 50 Times," Sun (UK), February 17, 2007, available at http://www.thesun.co.uk/sol/homepage/news/article18481.ece as of July 9, 2009.

302   "Age-Related Macular Degeneration," Resource Guide, National Eye Institute, U.S. National Institutes of Health, December 2007, available at http://www.nei.nih.gov/health/maculardegen/armd_facts.asp as of July 9, 2009.

303   Ibid; "RNIB Response to Statement by Nuffield Hospitals (re Leslie Howard)," Royal National Institute of Blind People (London, UK), April 24, 2007, available at http://www.rnib.org.uk/xpedio/groups/public/documents/PublicWebsite/public_pr250407.hcsp as of July 9, 2009.

304   Mark Branagan, "Pensioner is Refused Sight Drugs – Until He Goes Blind," Yorkshire Post (UK), April 24, 2007, available at http://www.yorkshirepost.co.uk/news?articleid=2724719 as of July 9, 2009.

305   Ibid; Paul Jeeves, "Pensioner Attacks NHS as Free Treatment Starts," Yorkshire Post (UK), May 1, 2007, available at http://www.yorkshirepost.co.uk/news/Pensioner-attacks-NHS--as.2842504.jp as of July 9, 2009.

306   "Man Must Go Blind to Get NHS Help," BBC News (UK), April 24, 2007, available at http://news.bbc.co.uk/2/hi/uk_news/england/north_yorkshire/6586785.stm as of July 9, 2009.

307   Ibid.

308   Ibid.

309   "OAP 'Must Go Blind to Get NHS Care,'" Daily Mail (UK), April 24, 2007, available at http://www.dailymail.co.uk/pages/live/articles/news/news.html?in_article_id=450309&in_page_id=1770&in_a_source=&ito=1490 as of July 9, 2009.

310   Paul Poutledge, "Oh Gord! Please Answer NHS.O.S.," Mirror (UK), April 27, 2007.

311   Paul Jeeves, "Pensioner Attacks NHS as Free Treatment Starts," Yorkshire Post (UK), May 1, 2007, available at http://www.yorkshirepost.co.uk/news/Pensioner-attacks-NHS--as.2842504.jp as of July 9, 2009.

312   Ibid.

313   "Eye Drug Decision is 'Long Overdue,'" Yorkshire Post (UK), April 2, 2008.

314   Paul Jeeves, "Pensioner Attacks NHS as Free Treatment Starts," Yorkshire Post (UK), May 1, 2007, available at http://www.yorkshirepost.co.uk/news/Pensioner-attacks-NHS--as.2842504.jp as of July 9, 2009.

315   David Derbyshire, "Blindness Drug U-Turn," Daily Mail (UK), August 27, 2008.

316   "Vital Drug against Blindness to Be Made Available on NHS," Yorkshire Post (UK), April 2, 2008.

317   "Ex-Nurse of Hutton Rudby Denied New Cancer Drug," Evening Gazette (UK), November 14, 2007.

318   Margarette Driscoll, "Fighting Cancer and the 'Unjust' Health Service," Times (UK), February 3, 2008, available at http://www.timesonline.co.uk/tol/life_and_style/health/article3294447.ece as of May 28, 2009.

319   Chris Brooke, "NHS Tells Cancer Patient Her Care Will Stop if She Buys Extra Drugs," Daily Mail (UK), December 16, 2007, available at http://www.dailymail.co.uk/pages/live/articles/news/news.html?in_article_id=502664&in_page_id=1770 as of July 9, 2009.

320   Ibid.

321   Margarette Driscoll, "Fighting Cancer and the 'Unjust' Health Service," Times (UK), February 3, 2008, available at http://www.timesonline.co.uk/tol/life_and_style/health/article3294447.ece as of May 28, 2009.

322   Hannah Chapman, "Cancer Patient Hoping for Support in NHS Drugs Battle," Northern Echo (UK), December 17, 2007, available at http://www.thenorthernecho.co.uk/news/topstories/display.var.1908666.0.cancer_patient_hoping_for_support_in_nhs_drugs_battle.php as of December 20, 2007.

323   Chris Brooke, "NHS Tells Cancer Patient Her Care Will Stop if She Buys Extra Drugs," Daily Mail (UK), December 16, 2007, available at http://www.dailymail.co.uk/pages/live/articles/news/news.html?in_article_id=502664&in_page_id=1770 as of July 9, 2009.

324   Margarette Driscoll, "Fighting Cancer and the 'Unjust' Health Service," Times (UK), February 3, 2008, available at http://www.timesonline.co.uk/tol/life_and_style/health/article3294447.ece as of May 28, 2009.

325   Sarah Kate Templeton, "NHS Threat to Halt Care for Cancer Patient," Times (UK), December 16, 2007, available at http://www.timesonline.co.uk/tol/life_and_style/health/article3056691.ece as of May 28, 2009.

326   "Private Cancer Care Top-Up Banned," BBC News (UK), December 16, 2007, available at http://news.bbc.co.uk/1/hi/england/7147030.stm as of July 9, 2009.

327   Chris Brooke, "NHS Tells Cancer Patient Her Care Will Stop if She Buys Extra Drugs," Daily Mail (UK), December 16, 2007, available at http://www.dailymail.co.uk/pages/live/articles/news/news.html?in_article_id=502664&in_page_id=1770 as of July 9, 2009.

328   Sophie Borland, "NHS May Deny Care to Woman over Avastin," Telegraph (UK), December 17, 2007, available at http://www.telegraph.co.uk/news/main.jhtml?xml=/news/2007/12/17/ncancer417.xml as of July 9, 2009.

329   Sarah Kate Templeton, "NHS Threat to Halt Care for Cancer Patient," Times (UK), December 16, 2007, available at http://www.timesonline.co.uk/tol/life_and_style/health/article3056691.ece as of July 15, 2009.

330   Ibid.

331   Sophie Borland, "NHS May Deny Care to Woman over Avastin," Telegraph (UK), December 17, 2007, available at http://www.telegraph.co.uk/news/main.jhtml?xml=/news/2007/12/17/ncancer417.xml as of December 20, 2007.

332   Chris Brooke, "NHS Tells Cancer Patient Her Care Will Stop if She Buys Extra Drugs," Daily Mail (UK), December 16, 2007, available at http://www.dailymail.co.uk/pages/live/articles/news/news.html?in_article_id=502664&in_page_id=1770 as of July 9, 2009.

333   "Ex-Nurse of Hutton Rudby Denied New Cancer Drug," Evening Gazette (UK), November 14, 2007.

334   Chris Brooke, "NHS Tells Cancer Patient Her Care Will Stop if She Buys Extra Drugs," Daily Mail (UK), December 16, 2007, available at http://www.dailymail.co.uk/pages/live/articles/news/news.html?in_article_id=502664&in_page_id=1770 as of July 9, 2009.

335   "Ex-Nurse of Hutton Rudby Denied New Cancer Drug," Evening Gazette (UK), November 14, 2007.

336   Chris Brooke, "NHS Tells Cancer Patient Her Care Will Stop if She Buys Extra Drugs," Daily Mail (UK), December 16, 2007, available at http://www.dailymail.co.uk/pages/live/articles/news/news.html?in_article_id=502664&in_page_id=1770 as of July 9, 2009.

337   Hannah Chapman, "Cancer Patient Hoping for Support in NHS Drugs Battle," Northern Echo (UK), December 17, 2007, available at http://www.thenorthernecho.co.uk/news/topstories/display.var.1908666.0.cancer_patient_hoping_for_support_in_nhs_drugs_battle.php as of December 20, 2007.

338   Margarette Driscoll, "Fighting Cancer and the 'Unjust' Health Service," Times (UK), February 3, 2008, available at http://www.timesonline.co.uk/tol/life_and_style/health/article3294447.ece as of May 28, 2009.

339   Karol Sikora, "Cancer Patient Failed by NHS," Sun (UK), December 18, 2007, available at http://www.thesun.co.uk/sol/homepage/news/article594569.ece as of December 20, 2007.

340   Sarah-Kate Templeton, "NHS Threat to Halt Care for Cancer Patient," Times (UK), December 16, 2007, available at http://www.timesonline.co.uk/tol/life_and_style/health/article3056691.ece as of July 9, 2009.

341   Daniel Martin, "Cancer Patients Get Right to Buy 'Top-Up' Drugs," Daily Mail (UK), November 3, 2008, available at http://www.dailymail.co.uk/health/article-1082469/Cancer-patients-right-buy-drugs.html as of May 28, 2009; "Alan Johnson Statement in Full," BBC (UK), November 4, 2008, available at http://news.bbc.co.uk/1/hi/uk_politics/7709282.stm as of May 28, 2009.

342   Angela Cole, "Couple's Delight at 'Top Up' About Turn," Kent Messenger (UK), November 14, 2008.

343   Sarah-Kate Templeton, "Cancer Woman Runs Out of Time in NHS Battle," The Times (UK), January 27, 2008, available at http://www.timesonline.co.uk/tol/news/uk/health/article3257529.ece as of July 9, 2009.

344   "Traumatic Home Birth for Mum Told to Drive 30 Miles to Next Hospital," Daily Mail (UK), December 19, 2007, available at http://www.dailymail.co.uk/pages/live/articles/health/womenfamily.html?in_article_id=503407&in_page_id=1799 as of July 10, 2009.

345   Ibid.

346   Ibid.

347   Ibid.

348   "Fears over Maternity Closures," Eastern Daily Press (UK), December 19, 2007.

349   "Traumatic Home Birth for Mum Told to Drive 30 Miles to Next Hospital," Daily Mail (UK), December 19, 2007, available at http://www.dailymail.co.uk/pages/live/articles/health/womenfamily.html?in_article_id=503407&in_page_id=1799 as of July 10, 2009.

350 "Fears over Maternity Closures," Eastern Daily Press (UK), December 19, 2007.

351 Ibid.

352 Powlesd, Norwich Evening News (UK), February 16, 2009.

353 For all source material and references, see "98-Year-Old Stranded in Hospital for Eight Hours as Jobsworths Refuse to Climb 4in Step," Daily Mail (UK), January 1, 2008, available at http://www.dailymail.co.uk/pages/live/articles/news/news.html?in_article_id=505582&in_page_id=1770&ei=dlx7R5GNKIy4ygS82O29Dg as of July 10, 2009.

354 Martin Stote, "Mum Forced to Pay £21,000 for a Cancer Drug to Save Her Life," Daily Express (UK), January 10, 2008, available at http://www.express.co.uk/posts/view/30963/Mum-forced-to-pay-21-000-for-a-cancer-drug-to-save-her-life as of July 8, 2009.

355 Ibid; "Woman Beats 'Terminal' Cancer after Funding Her Own Treatment," Daily Mail (UK), January 8, 2008, available at http://www.dailymail.co.uk/pages/live/articles/health/healthmain.html?in_article_id=507030&in_page_id=1774 as of January 15, 2008.

356 Emma Cullwick, "I Bought Lifesaver," Birmingham Evening Mail (UK), January 10, 2008, available at http://www.apria.com/resources/1,2725,494-709819,00.html as of January 15, 2008.

357 "Woman Beats 'Terminal' Cancer after Funding Her Own Treatment," Daily Mail (UK), January 8, 2008, available at http://www.dailymail.co.uk/pages/live/articles/health/healthmain.html?in_article_id=507030&in_page_id=1774 as of January 15, 2008.

358 Martin Stote, "Mum Forced to Pay £21,000 for a Cancer Drug to Save Her Life," Daily Express (UK), January 10, 2008, available at http://www.express.co.uk/posts/view/30963/Mum-forced-to-pay-21-000-for-a-cancer-drug-to-save-her-life as of July 8, 2009; Tom Rayner, "Campaigning Cancer Patient's Family 'Thrilled,'" Press Association Newsfile, November 4, 2008.

359 Sophie Borland, "NHS May Deny Care to Woman over Avastin," Telegraph (UK), December 17, 2007, available at http://www.telegraph.co.uk/news/main.jhtml?xml=/news/2007/12/17/ncancer417.xml as of June 1, 2009.

360 Ibid; Laura Donnelly, "NHS's Refusal to Fund Cancer Treatment Costs Mother £21,000," Telegraph (UK), September 14, 2008, available at http://www.telegraph.co.uk/health/2910780/NHSs-refusal-to-fund-cancer-treatment-costs-mother-21000.html as of June 1, 2009.

361 "Woman Beats 'Terminal' Cancer after Funding Her Own Treatment," Daily Mail (UK), January 8, 2008, available at http://www.dailymail.co.uk/pages/live/articles/health/healthmain.html?in_article_id=507030&in_page_id=1774 as of January 15, 2008.

362 Ibid.

363 Ibid.

364 Ibid.

365 Emma Cullwick, "Mum Defies NHS Medics' Gloomy Prognosis and Pays for Miracle Drug," Birmingham Mail (UK), January 10, 2008, available at http://www.apria.com/common/aw_cmp_printNews/1,2762,709819,00.html as of January 15, 2008.

366 "Woman Beats 'Terminal' Cancer after Funding Her Own Treatment," Daily Mail (UK), January 8, 2008, available at http://www.dailymail.co.uk/pages/live/articles/health/healthmain.html?in_article_id=507030&in_page_id=1774 as of January 15, 2008.

367 James Connell, "'Miracle' Cancer Drug Won't Go on NHS," Worcester News (UK), April 8, 2008, available at http://www.worcesternews.co.uk/news/2181411.miracle_cancer_drug_wont_go_on_nhs/ as of June 1, 2009.

368 Tom Rayner, "Campaigning Cancer Patient's Family 'Thrilled,'" Press Association Newsfile, November 4, 2008.

369 "Top-Up Ban Lifted," Business Monitor International, December 1, 2008.

370 See Paul Britton, "Sex-Change Tattoo Op on NHS," Manchester Evening News (UK), April 19, 2006, available at http://www.manchestereveningnews.co.uk/news/health/s/211/211096_sexchange_tattoo_op_on_nhs.html as of July 16, 2009; Fionnuala Bourke, "NHS Spends Pounds 8 Million Removing Tattoos," Sunday Mercury (UK), October 29, 2006.

371 Unless otherwise noted, for all source material and references, see "War Veteran Let Down by NHS," Evening Star (UK), January 12, 2008.

372 See also Laura Donnelly," NHS Patients Wait Years for Hearing Aids," Telegraph (UK), December 31, 2007, available at http://www.telegraph.co.uk/news/main.jhtml?xml=/news/2007/12/30/nhear130.xml as of July 10, 2009.

373 Ibid.

374 "Briton Travels All the Way to India for Low-Cost Surgery," Agence France Presse, July 10, 2004; "If you Needed an Operation, Would you Rather Join the Queue Here in Britain – or Get the Job Done in India and Make a Holiday of It?," Independent (UK), August 9, 2004, available at http://news.independent.co.uk/health/article50871.ece as of January 25, 2008.

375   "If You Needed an Operation, Would You Rather Join the Queue Here in Britain – or Get the Job Done in India and Make a Holiday of It?," Independent (UK), August 9, 2004, available at http://news.independent.co.uk/health/article50871. ece as of July 10, 2009.

376   "Briton Travels All the Way to India for Low-Cost Surgery," Agence France Presse, July 10, 2004; David Callaghan, "Patient Goes to India to Avoid NHS Wait," Guardian (UK), July 9, 2004, available at http://www.guardian.co.uk/society/2004/jul/09/medicineandhealth.lifeandhealth as of January 25, 2008.

377   "Indian Op Woman Dodges NHS Wait," BBC News (UK), September 7, 2004, available at http://news.bbc.co.uk/1/hi/health/3879371.stm as of July 10, 2009.

378   "If you Needed an Operation, Would You Rather Join the Queue Here in Britain – or Get the Job Done in India and Make a Holiday of It?," Independent (UK), August 9, 2004, available at http://news.independent.co.uk/health/article50871. ece as of July 10, 2009.

379   Ibid.

380   "Indian Op Woman Dodges NHS Wait," BBC News (UK), September 7, 2004, available at http://news.bbc.co.uk/1/hi/health/3879371.stm as of July 10, 2009.

381   "If You Needed an Operation, Would You Rather Join the Queue Here in Britain – or Get the Job Done in India and Make a Holiday of It?," Independent (UK), August 9, 2004, available at http://news.independent.co.uk/health/article50871. ece as of July 10, 2009.

382   "Indian Op Woman Dodges NHS Wait," BBC News (UK), September 7, 2004, available at http://news.bbc.co.uk/1/hi/health/3879371.stm as of July 10, 2009.

383   "If You Needed an Operation, Would You Rather Join the Queue Here in Britain – or Get the Job Done in India and Make a Holiday of It?," Independent (UK), August 9, 2004, available at http://news.independent.co.uk/health/article50871. ece as of July 10, 2009.

384   Ibid.

385   Ibid.

386   "Record Numbers Go Abroad for Health Treatment with 70,000 Escaping NHS," Daily Mail (UK), October 28, 2007, available at http://www.dailymail.co.uk/pages/live/articles/news/news.html?in_article_id=490233 as of July 10, 2009; Patrick Sawer and Laura Donnelly, "Fears and Frustrations Driving Patients Abroad," Telegraph (UK), October 29, 2007, available at http://www.telegraph.co.uk/news/main.jhtml?xml=/news/2007/10/28/nhealth228.xml as of July 10, 2009.

387   Martin McKeown, "More Tourists Opt for a New Face in the Sun," Express (UK), April 13, 2008.

388   For all source material and references, unless otherwise noted, see Patricia Balsom, "Diary of My Final Days," Independent (UK), November 16, 2006, available at http://www.independent.co.uk/arts-entertainment/books/features/patricia-balsom-diary-of-my-final-days-424518.html as of July 10, 2009.

389   Maxine Frith, "Patricia Balsom, NHS Campaigner, Loses Battle for Life," Independent (UK), November 18, 2006, available at http://www.independent.co.uk/life-style/health-and-families/health-news/patricia-balsom-nhs-campaigner-loses-battle-for-life-424762.html as of July 10, 2009.

390   The Care Quality Commission replaced the Healthcare Commission in April 2009.

391   Rebecca Smith, "NHS Patients Face Humiliating Treatment," Telegraph (UK), May 12, 2008, available at http://www.telegraph.co.uk/news/main.jhtml?xml=/news/2007/12/05/nhs105.xml as of July 9, 2009.

392   Kate Devlin, "Hospitals Face Fines for Treating Patients on Mixed-Sex Wards, Says Alan Johnson," Telegraph (UK), January 28, 2009, available at http://www.telegraph.co.uk/health/healthnews/4373128/Hospitals-face-fines-for-treating-patients-on-mixed-sex-wards-says-Alan-Johnson.html as of July 10, 2009.

393   For all source material and references, unless otherwise noted, see "Couple Lodge Complaint over Cancelled Op," Evening Star (UK), April 11, 2007.

394   "How the NHS Works," National Health Service, 2007.

395   For all source material and references, unless otherwise noted, see Ben Guy, "Man Left in Agony for Eight Hours," Journal (UK), Feb. 16, 2008, available at http://www.journallive.co.uk/north-east-news/todays-news/tm_headline=man-left-in-agony-for-eight-hours%26method=full%26objectid=20483323%26print_version=1%26siteid=61634-name_page.html as of July 15, 2009.

396   Lucy Cockcroft, "A&E Patients 'Left in Ambulances for Hours,'" Telegraph (UK), February 17, 2008, available at http://www.telegraph.co.uk/news/main.jhtml?xml=/news/2008/02/18/nhealth218.xml as of July 15, 2009.

397   Ibid; Sam Oestreicher of Unison in Daniel Martin, "A&E Patients Left in Ambulances for up to Five Hours 'So Trusts can Meet Government Targets,'" Daily Mail (UK), February 18, 2008, available at http://www.dailymail.co.uk/pages/live/articles/news/news.html?in_article_id=515332&in_page_id=1770 as of July 15, 2009.

398   Attributable to Sam Oestreicher in Daniel Martin, "A&E Patients Left in Ambulances for up to Five Hours 'So Trusts can Meet Government Targets,'" Daily Mail (UK), February 18, 2008, available at http://www.dailymail.co.uk/pages/live/articles/news/news.html?in_article_id=515332&in_page_id=1770 as of July 15, 2009.

399   Lucy Cockcroft, "A&E Patients 'Left in Ambulances for Hours,'" Telegraph (UK), February 17, 2008, available at http://www.telegraph.co.uk/news/main.jhtml?xml=/news/2008/02/18/nhealth218.xml as of July 15, 2009.

400   Sarah Lyall, "Paying Patients Test British Health Care System," New York Times, February 21, 2008, available at http://www.nytimes.com/2008/02/21/world/europe/21britain.html?_r=1&pagewanted=print&oref=slogin as of July 15, 2009.

401   Amanda Crook, "Woman's Cancer Drug Dilemma," Manchester Evening News (UK), December 24, 2007, available at http://www.manchestereveningnews.co.uk/news/health/s/1029646_womans_cancer_drug_dilemma as of July 15, 2009.

402   "Cancer Woman in Drugs Fight Wins," BBC News (UK), February 2, 2008, available at http://news.bbc.co.uk/1/hi/england/cornwall/7224157.stm as of July 15, 2009.

403   Ibid.

404   Sarah Lyall, "Paying Patients Test British Health Care System," New York Times, February 21, 2008, available at http://www.nytimes.com/2008/02/21/world/europe/21britain.html?_r=1&pagewanted=print&oref=slogin as of July 15, 2009.

405   Graham Satchell, "'I Have Been Denied Vital Cancer Drug,'" BBC News (UK), January 1, 2008, available at http://news.bbc.co.uk/1/hi/health/7219373.stm as of July 15, 2009.

406   Sarah Lyall, "Paying Patients Test British Health Care System," New York Times, February 21, 2008, available at http://www.nytimes.com/2008/02/21/world/europe/21britain.html?_r=1&pagewanted=print&oref=slogin as of July 15, 2009.

407   Graham Satchell, "'I Have Been Denied Vital Cancer Drug,'" BBC News (UK), January 1, 2008, available at http://news.bbc.co.uk/1/hi/health/7219373.stm as of July 15, 2009.

408   Don Frame, "Cancer Victim's NHS Victory," Manchester Evening News (UK), February 5, 2008, available at http://www.manchestereveningnews.co.uk/news/health/s/1035162_cancer_victims_nhs_victory as of July 15, 2009.

409   Amanda Crook, "Woman's Cancer Drug Dilemma," Manchester Evening News (UK), December 24, 2007, available at http://www.manchestereveningnews.co.uk/news/health/s/1029646_womans_cancer_drug_dilemma as of July 15, 2009.

410   Sarah Lyall, "Paying Patients Test British Health Care System," New York Times, February 21, 2008, available at http://www.nytimes.com/2008/02/21/world/europe/21britain.html?_r=1&pagewanted=print&oref=slogin as of July 15, 2009.

411   Amanda Crook, "Woman's Cancer Drug Dilemma," Manchester Evening News (UK), December 24, 2007, available at http://www.manchestereveningnews.co.uk/news/health/s/1029646_womans_cancer_drug_dilemma as of July 15, 2009.

412   Graham Satchell, "'I Have Been Denied Vital Cancer Drug,'" BBC News (UK), January 1, 2008, available at http://news.bbc.co.uk/1/hi/health/7219373.stm as of July 15, 2009.

413   Sarah Lyall, "Paying Patients Test British Health Care System," New York Times, February 21, 2008, available at http://www.nytimes.com/2008/02/21/world/europe/21britain.html?_r=1&pagewanted=print&oref=slogin as of July 15, 2009.

414   Ibid.

415   Don Frame, "Cancer Victim's NHS Victory," Manchester Evening News (UK), February 5, 2008, available at http://www.manchestereveningnews.co.uk/news/health/s/1035162_cancer_victims_nhs_victory as of July 15, 2009.

416   Sarah Lyall, "Paying Patients Test British Health Care System," New York Times, February 21, 2008, available at http://www.nytimes.com/2008/02/21/world/europe/21britain.html?_r=1&pagewanted=print&oref=slogin as of July 15, 2009; "Cancer Patient Hits out over Care," BBC News (UK), December 19, 2007, available at http://news.bbc.co.uk/1/hi/england/cornwall/7151328.stm as of July 15, 2009.

417   Ibid.

418   "Cancer Patient Hits out over Care," BBC News (UK), December 19, 2007, available at http://news.bbc.co.uk/1/hi/england/cornwall/7151328.stm as of February 27, 2007.

419   Amanda Crook, "Woman's Cancer Drug Dilemma," Manchester Evening News (UK), December 24, 2007, available at http://www.manchestereveningnews.co.uk/news/health/s/1029646_womans_cancer_drug_dilemma as of July 15, 2009.

420   "U-Turn over Patients' Rights to 'Top Up' NHS Care," Western Morning News (UK), June 20, 2008.

421   Sarah Lyall, "Paying Patients Test British Health Care System," New York Times, February 21, 2008, available at http://www.nytimes.com/2008/02/21/world/europe/21britain.html?_r=1&pagewanted=print&oref=slogin as of July 15, 2009; "Cancer Woman in Drugs Fight Wins," BBC News (UK), February 2, 2008, available at http://news.bbc.co.uk/1/hi/england/cornwall/7224157.stm as of July 15, 2009.

422   "Cancer Woman in Drugs Fight Wins," BBC News (UK), February 2, 2008, available at http://news.bbc.co.uk/1/hi/england/cornwall/7224157.stm as of July 15, 2009.

423   Don Frame, "Cancer Victim's NHS Victory," Manchester Evening News (UK), February 5, 2008, available at http://www.manchestereveningnews.co.uk/news/health/s/1035162_cancer_victims_nhs_victory as of July 15, 2009.

424   Ibid.

425   "Top-Up Ban Lifted," Business Monitor International, December 1, 2008.

426   Chris Brooke, "Doctors Save Baby when Mother-to-Be Drowns in Bath after Nurses Ignore Fainting Warning," Daily Mail (UK), February 27, 2008, available at http://www.dailymail.co.uk/pages/live/articles/news/news.html?in_article_id=520672&in_page_id=1770 as of July 15, 2009.

427   Hellen Mullins, "Inquest Hears of Worksop Woman's Death in Town Maternity Unit," Worksop Guardian (UK), February 26, 2008, cached version available at http://64.233.169.104/search?q=cache:SxduSHqsO-8J:www.worksopguardian.co.uk/news/Inquest-hears-of-Worksop-woman39s.3816878.jp+lorraine+maddi+lack+of+oxygen+to+the+brain&hl=en&ct=clnk&cd=2&gl=us&client=safari as of July 12, 2009.

428   Chris Brooke, "Doctors Save Baby when Mother-to-Be Drowns in Bath after Nurses Ignore Fainting Warning," Daily Mail (UK), February 27, 2008, available at http://www.dailymail.co.uk/pages/live/articles/news/news.html?in_article_id=520672&in_page_id=1770 as of July 15, 2009.

429   Stephen Adams, "Midwives 'Left Woman to Drown in the Bath,'" Telegraph (UK), February 27, 2008, available at http://www.telegraph.co.uk/news/main.jhtml?xml=/news/2008/02/27/npregnant127.xml as of July 15, 2009.

430   Chris Brooke, "Doctors Save Baby when Mother-to-Be Drowns in Bath after Nurses Ignore Fainting Warning," Daily Mail (UK), February 27, 2008, available at http://www.dailymail.co.uk/pages/live/articles/news/news.html?in_article_id=520672&in_page_id=1770 as of July 15, 2009.

431   Ibid.

432   Lucy Bannerman, "Husband to Sue after Wife Drowned in Hospital Bath," Times (UK), February 27, 2008, available at http://www.timesonline.co.uk/tol/life_and_style/health/article3448450.ece as of July 15, 2009.

433   Chris Brooke, "Doctors Save Baby when Mother-to-Be Drowns in Bath after Nurses Ignore Fainting Warning," Daily Mail (UK), February 27, 2008, available at http://www.dailymail.co.uk/pages/live/articles/news/news.html?in_article_id=520672&in_page_id=1770 as of July 15, 2009.

434   Ibid.

435   Lucy Bannerman, "Husband to Sue after Wife Drowned in Hospital Bath," Times (UK), February 27, 2008, available at http://www.timesonline.co.uk/tol/life_and_style/health/article3448450.ece as of July 15, 2009.

436   Ibid; Stephen Adams, "Midwives 'Left Woman to Drown in the Bath,'" Telegraph (UK), February 27, 2008, available at http://www.telegraph.co.uk/news/main.jhtml?xml=/news/2008/02/27/npregnant127.xml as of July 15, 2009; Chris Brooke, "Doctors Save Baby when Mother-to-Be Drowns in Bath after Nurses Ignore Fainting Warning," Daily Mail (UK), February 27, 2008, available at http://www.dailymail.co.uk/pages/live/articles/news/news.html?in_article_id=520672&in_page_id=1770 as of July 15, 2009.

437   Stephen Adams, "Midwives 'Left Woman to Drown in the Bath,'" Telegraph (UK), February 27, 2008, available at http://www.telegraph.co.uk/news/main.jhtml?xml=/news/2008/02/27/npregnant127.xml as of July 15, 2009.

438   Lucy Bannerman, "Husband to Sue after Wife Drowned in Hospital Bath," Times (UK), February 27, 2008, available at http://www.timesonline.co.uk/tol/life_and_style/health/article3448450.ece as of July 15, 2009.

439   Debbie Lockett, "Husband of Tragic Worksop Mum Speaks out," Worksop Guardian (UK), February 27, 2008, available at http://www.worksopguardian.co.uk/news/Husband-of-tragic-Worksop-mum.3820648.jp as of July 15, 2009.

440   Ibid.

441   Arthur Martin, "Father Delivered Baby after Partner was Turned away from NHS Hospital – TWICE," Daily Mail (UK), October 18, 2007, available at http://www.dailymail.co.uk/pages/live/articles/news/news.html?in_article_id=488142 as of July 10, 2009.

442   Jayne Isaac, "Hospital Horror for Woman Forced to Give Birth at Home," Glamorgan Gazette (UK), October 1, 2007, available at http://icwales.icnetwork.co.uk/news/south-wales-news/bridgend-maesteg/tm_headline=hospital-horror-for-woman-forced-to-give-birth-at-home%26method=full%26objectid=19966127%26print_version=1%26siteid=91466-name_page.html as of October 19, 2007.

443   Laura Wright, "Dad Forced to Deliver Baby at Home," South Walkes Echo (UK), October 17, 2007, available at http://icwales.icnetwork.co.uk/news/cardiff-news/tm_headline=dad-forced-to-deliver-baby-at-home%26method=full%26objectid=19964360%26print_version=1%26siteid=91466-name_page.html as of October 19, 2007.

444   Arthur Martin, "Father Delivered Baby after Partner was Turned away from NHS Hospital – TWICE," Daily Mail (UK), October 18, 2007, available at http://www.dailymail.co.uk/pages/live/articles/news/news.html?in_article_id=488142 as of July 10, 2009.

445   Jayne Isaac, "Hospital Horror for Woman Forced to Give Birth at Home," Glamorgan Gazette (UK), October 1, 2007, available at http://icwales.icnetwork.co.uk/news/south-wales-news/bridgend-maesteg/tm_headline=hospital-horror-for-woman-forced-to-give-birth-at-home%26method=full%26objectid=19966127%26print_version=1%26siteid=91466-name_page.html as of October 19, 2007.

446   Arthur Martin, "Father Delivered Baby after Partner was Turned away from NHS Hospital – TWICE," Daily Mail (UK), October 18, 2007, available at http://www.dailymail.co.uk/pages/live/articles/news/news.html?in_article_id=488142 as of October 19, 2007.

447   Jayne Isaac, "Hospital Horror for Woman Forced to Give Birth at Home," Glamorgan Gazette (UK), October 1, 2007, available at http://icwales.icnetwork.co.uk/news/south-wales-news/bridgend-maesteg/tm_headline=hospital-horror-for-woman-forced-to-give-birth-at-home%26method=full%26objectid=19966127%26print_version=1%26siteid=91466-name_page.html as of July 10, 2009.

448   Ibid.

449   Arthur Martin, "Father Delivered Baby after Partner was Turned away from NHS Hospital – TWICE," Daily Mail (UK), October 18, 2007, available at http://www.dailymail.co.uk/pages/live/articles/news/news.html?in_article_id=488142 as of July 10, 2009.

450   Ibid; Laura Wright, "Dad Forced to Deliver Baby at Home," South Wales Echo (UK), October 17, 2007, available at http://icwales.icnetwork.co.uk/news/cardiff-news/tm_headline=dad-forced-to-deliver-baby-at-home%26method=full%26objectid=19964360%26print_version=1%26siteid=91466-name_page.html as of July 10, 2009.

451   Arthur Martin, "Father Delivered Baby after Partner was Turned away from NHS Hospital – TWICE," Daily Mail (UK), October 18, 2007, available at http://www.dailymail.co.uk/pages/live/articles/news/news.html?in_article_id=488142 as of July 10, 2009.

452   Ibid.

453   Ibid.

454   Jayne Isaac, "Hospital Horror for Woman Forced to Give Birth at Home," Glamorgan Gazette (UK), October 1, 2007, available at http://icwales.icnetwork.co.uk/news/south-wales-news/bridgend-maesteg/tm_headline=hospital-horror-for-woman-forced-to-give-birth-at-home%26method=full%26objectid=19966127%26print_version=1%26siteid=91466-name_page.html as of July 10, 2009.

455   Arthur Martin, "Father Delivered Baby after Partner was Turned away from NHS Hospital – TWICE," Daily Mail (UK), October 18, 2007, available at http://www.dailymail.co.uk/pages/live/articles/news/news.html?in_article_id=488142 as of July 10, 2009.

456   Ibid.

457   Jayne Isaac, "Hospital Horror for Woman Forced to Give Birth at Home," Glamorgan Gazette (UK), October 1, 2007, available at http://icwales.icnetwork.co.uk/news/south-wales-news/bridgend-maesteg/tm_headline=hospital-horror-for-woman-forced-to-give-birth-at-home%26method=full%26objectid=19966127%26print_version=1%26siteid=91466-name_page.html as of July 10, 2009.

458   Arthur Martin, "Father Delivered Baby after Partner was Turned away from NHS Hospital – TWICE," Daily Mail (UK), October 18, 2007, available at http://www.dailymail.co.uk/pages/live/articles/news/news.html?in_article_id=488142 as of July 10, 2009.

459   Bob Phillipson and Peder Clark, "Too Little, Too Late," BLISS, October 2007, p. 10.

460   Ibid.

461   Unless otherwise noted, for all source material and references see Greg Tindle, "24-Hour Hospital Bed Wait for OAP," South Wales Echo (UK), January 30, 2008, available at http://icwales.icnetwork.co.uk/news/cardiff-news/2008/01/30/24-hour-hospital-bed-wait-for-oap-91466-20412167/ as of July 10, 2009.

462   "Time Spent in NHS Wales Accident and Emergency Departments: December 2008," Welsh Assembly Government Health Statistics and Analysis Unit, January 22, 2009, p. 1, available at http://wales.gov.uk/docs/statistics/2009/090122sdr82009en.pdf?lang=en as of July 10, 2009.

463   Ibid., p. 2.

464   "A&E Patient Stuck on Trolley 'All Night,'" South Wales Evening Post (UK), November 19, 2007.

465   Ibid.

466 Ibid.

467 Ibid.

468 "All Night on a Trolley – and Still No Answers," South Wales Evening Post (UK), January 7, 2008.

469 Ibid.

470 Ibid; "Student's 10-Hour Trolley Wait," South Wales Evening Post (UK), January 3, 2008.

471 "Student's 10-Hour Trolley Wait," South Wales Evening Post (UK), January 3, 2008.

472 "All Night on a Trolley – and Still No Answers," South Wales Evening Post (UK), January 7, 2008.

473 Ibid.

474 Ibid.

475 "Student's 10-Hour Trolley Wait," South Wales Evening Post (UK), January 3, 2008.

476 "All Night on a Trolley – and Still No Answers," South Wales Evening Post (UK), January 7, 2008.

477 Ibid.

478 Ibid.

479 "Student's 10-Hour Trolley Wait," South Wales Evening Post (UK), January 3, 2008.

480 For all source material, see "Drama as Elderly Woman Screamed in Pain," Aberdeen Press and Journal (UK), September 25, 2007.

481 Simon Johnson and Craig Walker, "Patient Left on Hospital Floor for Four Hours," Aberdeen Evening Express (UK), May 23, 2006.

482 Frank Urquhart, "Outrage as Man, 88, Left Lying on Hospital Floor for Four Hours," Scotsman (UK), May 24, 2006.

483 Annie Brown, "Tears, Jeers, Double Lives and Scandal," Daily Record (UK), December 28, 2006.

484 Simon Johnson and Craig Walker, "Patient Left on Hospital Floor for Four Hours," Aberdeen Evening Express (UK), May 23, 2006.

485 Ibid.

486 Frank Urquhart, "Outrage as Man, 88, Left Lying on Hospital Floor for Four Hours," Scotsman (UK), May 24, 2006.

487 Ibid.

488 Simon Johnson, "'NHS Chief Washed Hands of My Dad's Hospital Fall,'" Aberdeen Evening Express (UK), May 26, 2006.

489 Frank Urquhart, "Outrage as Man, 88, Left Lying on Hospital Floor for Four Hours," Scotsman (UK), May 24, 2006.

490 Simon Johnson, "Ambulance Workers Defend Fall Man Delay," Aberdeen Evening Express (UK), May 24, 2006.

491 Frank Urquhart, "Outrage as Man, 88, Left Lying on Hospital Floor for Four Hours," Scotsman (UK), May 24, 2006.

492 Lindsay McIntosh, "Fall Patient was Victim of 'Rules over Basic Humanity,'" Aberdeen Press and Journal (UK), May 24, 2006.

493 Simon Johnson, "Ambulance Workers Defend Fall Man Delay," Aberdeen Evening Express (UK), May 24, 2006.

494 Simon Johnson and Craig Walker, "Patient Left on Hospital Floor for Four Hours," Aberdeen Evening Express (UK), May 23, 2006.

495 Ibid.

496 Frank Urquhart, "Outrage as Man, 88, Left Lying on Hospital Floor for Four Hours," Scotsman (UK), May 24, 2006

497 For all source material and references, see Mark McLaughlin, "Angry Mother Tells of Girl's Hospital Ordeal," Scotland Courier (UK), September 29, 2007, available at http://www.thecourier.co.uk/output/2007/09/29/newsstory1034902t0.asp as of August 17, 2009.

CANADA

1   Lee Greenberg, "Waiting Lists Drive Retiree to Rights Fight," Ottawa Citizen (Canada), May 3, 2007, p. A3; Kevin Steel, "A Stroke of Luck," Western Standard (Canada), December 4, 2006, p. 19.

2   "Real Health Care," Ottawa Citizen, May 4, 2007, p. F4.

3   Lee Greenberg, "Waiting Lists Drive Retiree to Rights Fight," Ottawa Citizen (Canada), May 3, 2007, p. A3.

4   Windsor Star, "Ontario's Option," Windsor Star (Canada), May 4, 2007, p. A8; Kevin Steel, "A Stroke of Luck," Western Standard (Canada), December 4, 2006, p. 19.

5   Lee Greenberg, "Waiting Lists Drive Retiree to Rights Fight," Ottawa Citizen (Canada), May 3, 2007, p. A3.

6   Kevin Steel, "A Stroke of Luck," Western Standard (Canada), December 4, 2006, p. 19.

7   "Chaoulli Comes to Ontario," National Post (Canada), May 3, 2007, p. A18.

8   Lee Greenberg, "Waiting Lists Drive Retiree to Rights Fight," Ottawa Citizen (Canada), May 3, 2007, p. A3.

9   "Top Court Strikes Down Quebec Private Health-Care Ban," CBC News (Canada), June 9, 2005, available at http://www.cbc.ca/canada/story/2005/06/09/newscoc-health050609.html as of June 15, 2007; Sheryl Smolkin, "Jumping the Queue," Employee Benefits News (Canada), February 1, 2007.

10   "Winnipeg Activist for Poor, Inner-City Renewal Dies," CBC News (Canada), Nov. 11, 2006; Bob Holliday, "A Man Who Walked the Walk," Winnipeg Sun (Canada), November 16, 2006.

11   Chris Kitching, "He Made a Difference," Winnipeg Sun (Canada), November 12, 2006.

12   Ibid.

13   "Antipoverty Activist, 49, Dies in Winnipeg," The Globe and Mail (Canada), November 13, 2006.

14   Harry Lehotsky, "Free Medicare Nice, If You Can Get It," Winnipeg Sun (Canada), April 30, 2006.

15   Harry Lehotsky, "God Has Given Me More than I Deserved," Winnipeg Sun (Canada), May 21, 2006.

16   Harry Lehotsky, "Free Medicare Nice, If You Can Get It," Winnipeg Sun (Canada), April 30, 2006.

17   Ibid.

18   Ibid; Harry Lehotsky, "God Has Given Me More than I Deserved," Winnipeg Sun (Canada), May 21, 2006.

19   Harry Lehotsky, "Free Medicare Nice, If You Can Get It," Winnipeg Sun (Canada), April 30, 2006.

20   Harry Lehotsky, "Good Works, Good People Will Carry On," Winnipeg Sun (Canada), June 11, 2006.

21   Harry Lehotsky, "This Thanksgiving, I Choose to be Grateful," Winnipeg Sun (Canada), October 8, 2006.

22   Harry Lehotsky, "Good Works, Good People Will Carry On," Winnipeg Sun (Canada), June 11, 2006.

23   "Winnipeg Activist for Poor, Inner-City Renewal Dies," CBC News (Canada), Nov. 11, 2006.

24   "Governor General Announces New Appointments to the Order of Canada," Media and Public Information, Governor General of Canada, February 20, 2007, available at http://www.gg.ca/media/doc.asp?lang=e&DocID=4984 as of July 15, 2009.

25   Frank Landry, "B.C. Man Prepares to Sue," Winnipeg Sun (Canada), July 1, 2003.

26   "The Winnipeg Regional Health Authority Will Investigate Why a Woman Died while Waiting for Heart Surgery," Broadcast News, February 11, 2003.

27   Ibid; "Canadian Health-Care Critique Finds Fodder in Waiting Lines," Edmonton Journal (Canada), October 22, 2005.

28   Scott Edmonds, "Tories Hit Emotional Health Issue," Portage Daily Graphic (Canada), May 23, 2003.

29   Ibid.

30   Frank Landry, "Surgery Delay Alarm Raised," Winnipeg Sun (Canada), February 10, 2004.

31   Rochelle Squires, "Heart-Surgery Fears," Winnipeg Sun (Canada), February 13, 2007.

32   Frank Landry, "'Chomiak Must Go,'" Winnipeg Sun (Canada), February 22, 2003.

33   Ibid.

34   "Man Can't Get Vital Skull Replacement Surgery," Ontario New Democratic Party, January 17, 2006, available at http://ontariondp.com/node/10/print as of July 9, 2009.

35   Tanya Talaga and Robert Cribb, "Year-Long Wait for Skull Surgery," Toronto Star (Canada), May 22, 2007, available at http://www.thestar.com/article/216280 as of July 9, 2009; "Man's Surgery Successful, Full Recovery on the Way," Keep In Touch, Andrea Horwath Community Report, Spring 2006, p. 3; "Are Your Pets Getting Better Care than You?," CityNews (Canada), July 2, 2007, available at http://www.citynews.ca/news/news_12475.aspx as of July 9, 2009.

36   "Man Can't Get Vital Skull Replacement Surgery," Ontario New Democratic Party, January 17, 2006, available at http://ontariondp.com/node/10/print as of July 9, 2009.

37   Tanya Talaga and Robert Cribb, "Year-Long Wait for Skull Surgery," Toronto Star (Canada), May 22, 2007, available at http://www.thestar.com/article/216280 as of July 9, 2009; Ibid.

38   Tanya Talaga and Robert Cribb, "Year-Long Wait for Skull Surgery," Toronto Star (Canada), May 22, 2007, available at http://www.thestar.com/article/216280 as of July 9, 2009; "Man Can't Get Vital Skull Replacement Surgery," Ontario New Democratic Party, January 17, 2006, available at http://ontariondp.com/node/10/print as of July 9, 2009.

39   "Are Your Pets Getting Better Care than You?," CityNews (Canada), July 2, 2007, available at http://www.citynews.ca/news/news_12475.aspx as of August 10, 2007.

40   Tanya Talaga and Robert Cribb, "Year-Long Wait for Skull Surgery," Toronto Star (Canada), May 22, 2007, available at http://www.thestar.com/article/216280 as of July 9, 2009.

41   "Are Your Pets Getting Better Care than You?," CityNews (Canada), July 2, 2007, available at http://www.citynews.ca/news/news_12475.aspx as of July 9, 2009.

42   Tanya Talaga and Robert Cribb, "Year-Long Wait for Skull Surgery," Toronto Star (Canada), May 22, 2007, available at http://www.thestar.com/article/216280 as of July 9, 2009.

43   Ibid.

44   "Man Can't Get Vital Skull Replacement Surgery," Ontario New Democratic Party, January 17, 2006, available at http://ontariondp.com/node/10/print as of July 9, 2009.

45   "Man's Surgery Successful, Full Recovery on the Way," Keep In Touch, Andrea Horwath Community Report, Spring 2006, p. 3.

46   Tanya Talaga and Robert Cribb, "Year-Long Wait for Skull Surgery," Toronto Star (Canada), May 22, 2007, available at http://www.thestar.com/article/216280 as of July 9, 2009.

47   "Man Can't Get Vital Skull Replacement Surgery," Ontario New Democratic Party, January 17, 2006, available at http://ontariondp.com/node/10/print as of July 9, 2009.

48   Tanya Talaga and Robert Cribb, "Year-Long Wait for Skull Surgery," Toronto Star (Canada), May 22, 2007, available at http://www.thestar.com/article/216280 as of July 9, 2009.

49   Sarah Cooke, "Canadian Woman Delivers Rare Identical Quadruplets at Montana Hospital," Associated Press, August 17, 2007.

50   Unnati Gandhi, "Twins, Times Two, Born to Calgary Mother," Globe and Mail (Canada), August 17, 2007.

51   "Calgary Woman Delivers Rare Set of Identical Quadruplets in U.S. Hospital," Canadian Press NewsWire (Canada), August 6, 2007; "Calgary Woman Delivers Identical Quadruplets in U.S.," CBC News, August 16, 2007.

52   Unnati Gandhi, "Twins, Times Two, Born to Calgary Mother," Globe and Mail (Canada), August 17, 2007.

53   Ibid.

54   Ibid.

55   Michelle Lang and Keith Bonnell, "Identical Quadruplets 'Small, but Healthy,'" Ottawa Citizen (UK), August 17, 2007.

56   "Calgary Mother of Quads Thrilled, Overwhelmed," CBC News, August 21, 2007.

57   "Calgary Woman Delivers Rare Set of Identical Quadruplets in U.S. Hospital," Canadian Press NewsWire (Canada), August 6, 2007; Kristen Cates, "Four of a Kind," Great Falls Tribune, August 17, 2007.

58   Robin Roberts and Chris Cuomo, "Meet the Identical Quads," Good Morning America, ABC News, August 22, 2007.

59   Doug McIntyre, "Mom Has Identical Quads," Edmonton Sun (Canada), August 17, 2007.

60   Unnati Gandhi, "Twins, Times Two, Born to Calgary Mother," Globe and Mail (Canada), August 17, 2007.

61   Larry Pynn, "No Room in B.C., Preemie Twins Born in Alberta," Times Colonist (Canada), May 29, 2004; Mark Steyn, "Happy Warrior," National Review, July 4, 2005.

62   Larry Pynn and Chad Skelton, "No Hospital Beds in B.C., Mom-to-Be Flown to Alberta," Vancouver Sun (Canada), May 29, 2004.

63   Ibid.

64   Ibid.

65   Larry Pynn, "No Room in B.C., Preemie Twins Born in Alberta," Times Colonist (Canada), May 29, 2004.

66   Larry Pynn and Chad Skelton, "No Hospital Beds in B.C., Mom-to-Be Flown to Alberta," Vancouver Sun (Canada), May 29, 2004.

67   Ibid.

68   Ibid; Larry Pynn, "No Room in B.C., Preemie Twins Born in Alberta," Times Colonist (Canada), May 29, 2004.

69   Larry Pynn, "No Room in B.C., Preemie Twins Born in Alberta," Times Colonist (Canada), May 29, 2004.

70   "Ryan Gets His MRI, but Long Waiting Lists Remain," CBC News (Canada), February 3, 2005, available at http://www.cbc.ca/canada/newfoundland-labrador/story/2005/02/03/nf-mri-wait-20050203.html as of July 12, 2009.

71   "MRI Wait for Son Too Long, Mother Says," CBC News (Canada), January 13, 2005, available at http://www.cbc.ca/canada/newfoundland-labrador/story/2005/01/13/nf-mri-wait-20050112.html as of July 12, 2009.

72   Stokes Sullivan, "'Access Denied,'" St. John's Telegram (Canada), January 14, 2005.

73   Mayo Clinic Staff, "Wilms' Tumor," Mayo Foundation for Medical Education and Research, Rochester, MN, September 7, 2008, available at http://www.mayoclinic.com/print/wilms-tumor/DS00436/METHOD=print&DSECTION=1 as of July 12, 2009.

74   "MRI Wait for Son Too Long, Mother Says," CBC News (Canada), January 13, 2005, available at http://www.cbc.ca/canada/newfoundland-labrador/story/2005/01/13/nf-mri-wait-20050112.html as of July 12, 2009.

75   Lisa Priest, "A Boy's Plight, a Nation's Problem," Globe and Mail (Canada), January 13, 2005, available at http://www.liberty-page.com/issues/healthcare/canboysplight.html as of July 12, 2009.

76   This, according to Normand Laberge, CEO of the Canadian Association of Radiologists. "[Ryan Oldford] had to wait three or four months before the hospital called [to add him to the MRI wait list] March 26, 2008." Quoted in Stokes Sullivan, "'Access Denied,'" St. John's Telegram (Canada), January 14, 2005.

77   Lisa Priest, "A Boy's Plight, a Nation's Problem," Globe and Mail (Canada), January 13, 2005, available at http://www.liberty-page.com/issues/healthcare/canboysplight.html as of July 12, 2009.

78   Lisa Priest, "Newfoundland Boy who Needs MRI May Turn to U.S.," Globe and Mail (Canada), January 27, 2005.

79   "MRI Wait for Son Too Long, Mother Says," CBC News (Canada), January 13, 2005, available at http://www.cbc.ca/canada/newfoundland-labrador/story/2005/01/13/nf-mri-wait-20050112.html as of July 12, 2009.

80   Stokes Sullivan, "'Access Denied,'" St. John's Telegram (Canada), January 14, 2005.

81   Lisa Priest, "Newfoundland Boy who Needs MRI May Turn to U.S.," Globe and Mail (Canada), January 27, 2005.

82   Derek Hunter, "Doing Your Own Health Care Thing: American Seniors vs. Canadian Citizens," The Heritage Foundation, Washington, DC, July 1, 2005, available at http://www.heritage.org/Research/HealthCare/wm782.cfm as of July 12, 2009.

83   Lisa Priest, "Newfoundland Boy who Needs MRI May Turn to U.S.," Globe and Mail (Canada), January 27, 2005.

84   Ibid.

85   Ibid.

86   "Ryan Gets His MRI, but Long Waiting Lists Remain," CBC News (Canada), February 3, 2005, available at http://www.cbc.ca/canada/newfoundland-labrador/story/2005/02/03/nf-mri-wait-20050203.html as of July 12, 2009.

87   "Gander Gains Edge with New MRI Machine," CBC News (Canada), June 2, 2009, available at http://www.cbc.ca/canada/newfoundland-labrador/story/2009/06/02/gander-mri-602.html as of July 12, 2009.

88   "Quarterly Demographic Estimates," Statistics Canada, March 26, 2009, available at http://www.statcan.gc.ca/daily-quotidien/090326/t090326a2-eng.htm as of June 5, 2009.

89   Unless otherwise noted, for all source material and references, see Janet French, "Elderly Woman's Family Upset by Surgery Wait," StarPhoenix (Canada), November 9, 2007, available at http://www.canada.com/saskatoonstarphoenix/news/local/story.html?id=025e887a-e059-48c3-b885-0e535684a862 as of July 10, 2009.

90   Nadeem Esmail, "Hospital Waiting Lists in Canada," 17th edition, Fraser Institute (Canada), p. 3, available at http://www.fraserinstitute.org/Commerce.Web/product_files/wyt2007.pdf as of July 10, 2009.

91   Pamela Fayerman, "B.C. Patient Seeks Help with U.S. Bill," Vancouver Sun (Canada), November 27, 2006, available at http://www.canada.com/vancouversun/news/westcoastnews/story.html?id=272935e1-04fa-4bd8-ac41-8d6183d77c0b&p=1 as of July 9, 2009.

92   Ibid.

93   Randy Hall, "America Is Not 'Sicko,' Filmmaker to Tell Lawmakers," CNS News, June 21, 2007.

94   Pamela Fayerman, "B.C. Patient Seeks Help with U.S. Bill," Vancouver Sun (Canada), November 27, 2006, available at http://www.canada.com/vancouversun/news/westcoastnews/story.html?id=272935e1-04fa-4bd8-ac41-8d6183d77c0b&p=1 as of July 9, 2009.

95   Camille Jensen, "20/20 Visits Vernon," Castanet (Canada), August 20, 2007, available at http://www.castanet.net/edition/news-story-31988--search.htm as of July 9, 2009.

96   Sam Solomon, "Chaoulli Copycat Cases Crop Up Across Country," National Review of Medicine (Canada), Vol. 4, No. 1, January 15, 2007, available at http://www.nationalreviewofmedicine.com/issue/2007/01_15/4_policy_politics02_1.html as of July 9, 2009.

97   Pamela Fayerman, "B.C. Patient Seeks Help with U.S. Bill," Vancouver Sun (Canada), November 27, 2006, available at http://www.canada.com/vancouversun/news/westcoastnews/story.html?id=272935e1-04fa-4bd8-ac41-8d6183d77c0b&p=1 as of July 9, 2009.

98   Ibid.

99   John Carpay, "Taking Canada's Medical Monopolies to Court," Fraser Forum, Fraser Institute (Canada), February 2007, available at http://www.canadianconstitutionfoundation.ca/files/pdf/fraserforum-02-01-2007.pdf as of July 9, 2009.

100   Pamela Fayerman, "B.C. Patient Seeks Help with U.S. Bill," Vancouver Sun (Canada), November 27, 2006, available at http://www.canada.com/vancouversun/news/westcoastnews/story.html?id=272935e1-04fa-4bd8-ac41-8d6183d77c0b&p=1 as of July 9, 2009.

101   Kyle Harland, "Woman Suing to Recoup U.S. Medical Costs," Globe and Mail (Canada), November 23, 2007.

102   Camille Jensen, "20/20 Visits Vernon," Castanet (Canada), August 20, 2007, available at http://www.castanet.net/edition/news-story-31988--search.htm as of July 22, 2009.

103   "News," Timely Medical Alternatives (Vancouver, Canada), November 23, 2007, available at http://www.timelymedical.ca/news.html as of May 26, 2009.

104   Kyle Harland, "Woman Suing to Recoup U.S. Medical Costs," Globe and Mail (Canada), November 23, 2007.

105   Sam Solomon, "BC Patient-Cum-Plaintiff Shirley Healey Dies," Canadian Medicine blog, May 20, 2008, available at http://www.canadianmedicinenews.com/2008/05/bc-patient-cum-plaintiff-shirley-healey.html as of May 26, 2009.

106   Ibid.

107   "Healey Passes," AM 1150 (Canada), May 16, 2008, available at http://www.am1150.ca/news/565/720321 as of May 26, 2009.

108   Kelly Sinoski, "B.C. Patient Left Stranded in U.S. by Bed Shortage," Vancouver Sun (Canada), January 2, 2008, available at http://www.canada.com/vancouversun/news/story.html?id=41790c51-679c-4a22-8301-f1278e664ae6 as of July 10, 2009.

109   Ibid.

110   Ibid.

111   Ibid.

112   Ibid.

113   Jonathan Fowlie and Kelly Sinoski, "Bed Opens up in B.C. for Surrey Woman Stranded in California Hospital," Vancouver Sun (Canada), January 2, 2008, available at http://www.canada.com/vancouversun/news/story.html?id=b2594d00-d8a2-48e7-82d0-d2c4c56f12ca&k=56389 as of July 10, 2009.

114   For all source material and references, unless otherwise noted, see Laura Drake, "Hospital Had to Send Man to Montreal for Surgery," Ottawa Citizen (Canada), October 19, 2007, available at http://www.canada.com/ottawacitizen/news/story.html?id=bd7f6fd5-f4d1-4573-b298-305828f961b6&k=15068&p=1 as of March 12, 2008.

115   Laura Drake, "Appendix Removal Took 28 Hours," National Post (Canada), October 19, 2007.

116   Statistic cited in BMJ Best Treatments on Appendicitis, British Medical Journal Group, London, UK, September 27, 2007, available at http://besttreatments.bmj.com/btuk/conditions/1000083260.html#ref5 as of March 12, 2008.

117   John Miner, "Bed Shortage Nixes Teen's Life-Saving Heart Surgery," London Free Press (Canada), April 7, 2007, p. B1, available at http://www.lfpress.ca/cgi-bin/publish.cgi?p=178597&x=articles&s=health as of July 15, 2009.

118   Ibid.

119   Ibid.

120   Ibid.

121   John Miner, "Heart Surgery Cancelled Again," London Free Press (Canada), April 25, 2007, p. B5, available at http://lfpress.ca/cgi-bin/publish.cgi?p=180790&s=careers as of July 15, 2009.

122   Ibid.

123   For all source material and references, unless otherwise noted, see Doug Williamson, "Cancer Survivor Battles OHIP," Windsor Star (Canada), March 11, 2008, available at http://www.canada.com/windsorstar/news/story.html?id=3ccdf1b2-7409-40d2-8b80-55f3cdc441d0&k=82139 as of July 12, 2009.

124   Doug Williamson, "Smitherman Won't Intervene in Cancer Survivor's OHIP Battle," Windsor Star (Canada), March 12, 2008, available at http://www.canada.com/windsorstar/news/local/story.html?id=0246f064-9769-4c6e-951f-3ebf89f1f852&k=67053 as of July 12, 2009.

125   Ibid.

126   Peter Downs, "Skier Waits 4 Days for Surgery," St. Catherines Standard (Canada), February 28, 2008.

127   Telephone interview of Peter Downs, reporter for St. Catherines Standard, March 4, 2008.

128   Peter Downs, "Skier Waits 4 Days for Surgery," St. Catherines Standard (Canada), February 28, 2008.

129   Ibid.

130   Ibid.

131   Ibid.

132   "Injured St. Catherines Skier Finally Gets Her Operation," St. Catherines Standard (Canada), February 29, 2008.

133   Peter Downs, "Skier Waits 4 Days for Surgery," St. Catherines Standard (Canada), February 28, 2008.

134   Ibid.

135   Ibid.

136   Jason Fekete, "Ailing Albertans Seek Help Abroad," Calgary Herald (Canada), July 31, 2004.

137   Richard Brennan and Robert Benzie, "Countries Offer Quick Getaway from Waiting Lists," Toronto Star (Canada), September 11, 2004.

138   Jeremy Copeland, "Canadian Medical Tourists in India," CBC News (Canada), September 20, 2004, available at http://www.cbc.ca/news/viewpoint/vp_copeland/20040920.html as of July 15, 2009.

139   Ibid.

140   Jason Fekete, "Ailing Albertans Seek Help Abroad," Calgary Herald (Canada), July 31, 2004.

141   Jeremy Copeland, "Canadian Medical Tourists in India," CBC News (Canada), September 20, 2004, available at http://www.cbc.ca/news/viewpoint/vp_copeland/20040920.html as of July 15, 2009.

142   Richard Brennan and Robert Benzie, "Countries Offer Quick Getaway from Waiting Lists," Toronto Star (Canada), September 11, 2004.

143   Jeremy Copeland, "Canadian Medical Tourists in India," CBC News (Canada), September 20, 2004, available at http://www.cbc.ca/news/viewpoint/vp_copeland/20040920.html as of July 15, 2009.

144   Richard Brennan and Robert Benzie, "Countries Offer Quick Getaway from Waiting Lists," Toronto Star (Canada), September 11, 2004.

145   Ibid.

146   Jeremy Copeland, "Canadian Medical Tourists in India," CBC News (Canada), September 20, 2004, available at http://www.cbc.ca/news/viewpoint/vp_copeland/20040920.html as of July 15, 2009.

147   Ibid.

148   Richard Brennan and Robert Benzie, "Countries Offer Quick Getaway from Waiting Lists," Toronto Star (Canada), September 11, 2004.

149   Jason Fekete, "Ailing Albertans Seek Help Abroad," Calgary Herald (Canada), July 31, 2004.

150   Michelle Lang, "Calgarians Push for Costs on Cross-Border Surgery," Calgary Herald (Canada), August 1, 2005.

151   Nadeem Esmail and Michael Walker, "Waiting Your Turn," 17th Ed., The Fraser Institute (Canada), 2007, p. 15, available at http://www.fraserinstitute.org/COMMERCE.WEB/product_files/WaitingYourTurn2007rev2.pdf as of July 15, 2009.

152   Ibid., p. 7. Report cites Statistics Canada, 2005 data.

153   Peter Downs, "No Time to Wait," Standard (Canada), January 7, 2006.

154   Ibid.

155   Heather Sokoloff, "'How Much Do you Spend for an Extra Life?'" National Post (Canada), February 1, 2006.

156   Ibid.

157   Peter Downs, "Cancer Fighter Says 'Government's Letting Me Down,'" Standard (Canada), November 19, 2005.

158   Heather Sokoloff, "'How Much Do you Spend for an Extra Life?'" National Post (Canada), February 1, 2006.

159   Peter Downs, "Cancer Fighter Says 'Government's Letting Me Down,'" Standard (Canada), November 19, 2005.

160   Peter Downs, "No Time to Wait," Standard (Canada), January 7, 2006.

161   Trish Audette, "'I Know a Lot of People are Praying for Me,'" Standard (Canada), October 18, 2004.

162   Peter Downs, "Her Life, Her Story," Standard (Canada), November 12, 2007.

163   Peter Downs, "No Time to Wait," Standard (Canada), January 7, 2006.

164   Heather Sokoloff, "'How Much Do you Spend for an Extra Life?'" National Post (Canada), February 1, 2006.

165   Peter Downs, "Finding Hope after Reality's Harsh Return," Standard (Canada), February 14, 2006.

166   Peter Downs, "No Time to Wait," Standard (Canada), January 7, 2006.

167   Lisa Priest, "Ontario Changes Tack on Cancer Drugs," Globe and Mail (Canada), May 5, 2006.

168   Peter Downs, "Cancer Fighter Says 'Government's Letting Me Down,'" Standard (Canada), November 19, 2005.

169   Kelly Patrick, "'An Inefficient System,'" National Post (Canada), September 18, 2006.

170   Lisa Priest, "Ontario Changes Tack on Cancer Drugs," Globe and Mail (Canada), May 5, 2006.

171   Peter Downs, "'I Get Why People Go Postal Now,'" Standard (Canada), July 4, 2006.

172   Ibid.

173   Kelly Patrick, "'An Inefficient System,'" National Post (Canada), September 18, 2006.

174   Peter Downs, "Another Bureaucratic Battle Takes Its Toll," Standard (Canada), September 22, 2006.

175   Rob Ferguson, "Cancer Drug Claim Rejected by OHIP," Toronto Star (Canada), November 17, 2006.

176   Rob Ferguson, "Ontario to Pay $76,000 Bill," Toronto Star (Canada), January 31, 2007.

177   Peter Downs, "Victory for Suzanne," Standard (Canada), January 31, 2007.

178   Rob Ferguson, "Ontario to Pay $76,000 Bill," Toronto Star (Canada), January 31, 2007.

179   Peter Downs, "She Touched Us All," Standard (Canada), November 12, 2007.

180   For all source material and references, see Lisa Priest, "Long Wait Forces Cancer Patient to Buy Operation in Land He Fled," Globe and Mail (Canada), January 31, 2007, available at http://www.zavitzinsurance.com/documents/Globe-andMailCIPatient.pdf as of July 22, 2009.

181   Susan Warner, Radio Interview, "The Current," Canadian Broadcast Corporation (CBC), January 10, 2006, audio available at http://www.cbc.ca/thecurrent/2006/200601/20060110.html as of July 22, 2009.

182   Ibid.

183   Jason Fekete, "Need Surgery? Here's How Long you'll Wait," Calgary Herald (Canada), July 28, 2004, available at http://www.liberty-page.com/issues/healthcare/wait.html as of June 11, 2008.

184   Ibid.

185   Susan Warner, Radio Interview, "The Current," Canadian Broadcast Corporation (CBC), January 10, 2006, audio available at http://www.cbc.ca/thecurrent/2006/200601/20060110.html as of July 22, 2009.

186   Ibid.

187   Ibid.

188   Jason Fekete, "Need Surgery? Here's How Long you'll Wait," Calgary Herald (Canada), July 28, 2004, available at http://www.liberty-page.com/issues/healthcare/wait.html as of June 11, 2008.

189   Susan Warner, Radio Interview, "The Current," Canadian Broadcast Corporation (CBC), January 10, 2006, audio available at http://www.cbc.ca/thecurrent/2006/200601/20060110.html as of July 22, 2009.

190   Ibid.

191   Ibid.

192   Michelle Lang, "Surgery Wait Lists Four Times Too Long," Calgary Herald (Canada), March 1, 2005.

193   Brigitte Pellerin, "Viewer Discretion Is Advised," Western Standard (Canada), November 28, 2005.

194   Susan Warner, Radio Interview, "The Current," Canadian Broadcast Corporation (CBC), January 10, 2006, audio available at http://www.cbc.ca/thecurrent/2006/200601/20060110.html as of July 22, 2009.

195   "Wait List Insurance a Tough Sell among Medicare Supporters," Canadian Broadcast Corporation (CBC), May 20, 2008, available at http://www.cbc.ca/health/story/2008/05/20/wait-list.html?ref=rss as of June 11, 2008.

196   Susan Warner, Radio Interview, "The Current," Canadian Broadcast Corporation (CBC), January 10, 2006, audio available at http://www.cbc.ca/thecurrent/2006/200601/20060110.html as of July 22, 2009.

197   For all source material and references, see André Picard, "A Jaw-Dropping Wait Time for Surgery," Globe and Mail (Canada), May 22, 2007, last updated on March 31, 2009, available at http://www.theglobeandmail.com/servlet/story/RTGAM.20070522.wxljaw22/BNStory/specialScienceandHealth/home as of July 15, 2009.

198   Mary Caton, "'He's Going to Die if I Don't Do This,'" Windsor Star (Canada), December 5, 2007, available at http://www.canada.com/windsorstar/news/story.html?id=a567b53b-1b8e-4ab5-9fab-65666fe2457e as of June 23, 2009.

199   Meira Curley, Letter to Hon. George Smitherman, available at http://www.chadcurley.com/chad_curley.htm as of July 31, 2008.

200   Ibid.

201   Mary Caton, "'He's Going to Die if I Don't Do This,'" Windsor Star (Canada), December 5, 2007, available at http://www.canada.com/windsorstar/news/story.html?id=a567b53b-1b8e-4ab5-9fab-65666fe2457e as of June 23, 2009.

202   Meira Curley, Letter to Hon. George Smitherman, available at http://www.chadcurley.com/chad_curley.htm as of July 31, 2008.

203   Mary Caton, "'He's Going to Die if I Don't Do This,'" Windsor Star (Canada), December 5, 2007, available at http://www.canada.com/windsorstar/news/story.html?id=a567b53b-1b8e-4ab5-9fab-65666fe2457e as of June 23, 2009.

204   Ibid.

205   Meira Curley, Letter to Hon. George Smitherman, available at http://www.chadcurley.com/chad_curley.htm as of July 31, 2008.

206   Mary Caton, "'He's Going to Die if I Don't Do This,'" Windsor Star (Canada), December 5, 2007, available at http://www.canada.com/windsorstar/news/story.html?id=a567b53b-1b8e-4ab5-9fab-65666fe2457e as of June 23, 2009.

207   Meira Curley, Letter to Hon. George Smitherman, available at http://www.chadcurley.com/chad_curley.htm as of July 31, 2008.

208   Mary Caton, "'He's Going to Die if I Don't Do This,'" Windsor Star (Canada), December 5, 2007, available at http://www.canada.com/windsorstar/news/story.html?id=a567b53b-1b8e-4ab5-9fab-65666fe2457e as of July 31, 2008.

209   Meira Curley, Letter to Hon. George Smitherman, available at http://www.chadcurley.com/chad_curley.htm as of July 31, 2008.

210   Mary Caton, "'He's Going to Die if I Don't Do This,'" Windsor Star (Canada), December 5, 2007, available at http://www.canada.com/windsorstar/news/story.html?id=a567b53b-1b8e-4ab5-9fab-65666fe2457e as of June 23, 2009.

211   Robert M. Goldberg, "How 'Liberal' Care Would Kill Ted," New York Post, June 5, 2008, available at http://www.nypost.com/seven/06052008/postopinion/opedcolumnists/how_liberal_care_would_kill_ted_114032.htm as of July 22, 2009.

212   Meira Curley, Letter to Hon. George Smitherman, available at http://www.chadcurley.com/chad_curley.htm as of July 31, 2008.

213   Mary Caton, "'He's Going to Die if I Don't Do This,'" Windsor Star (Canada), December 5, 2007, available at http://www.canada.com/windsorstar/news/story.html?id=a567b53b-1b8e-4ab5-9fab-65666fe2457e as of June 23, 2009.

214   Ibid.

215   Ibid.

216   Meira Curley, Letter to Hon. George Smitherman, available at http://www.chadcurley.com/chad_curley.htm as of July 31, 2008.

217   See Photos of December 30, 2007 fundraiser at http://www.chadcurley.com/Fundraiser=20-=20Golf/INDEX.HTML as of July 31, 2008.

218   Meira Curley, Letter to Hon. George Smitherman, available at http://www.chadcurley.com/chad_curley.htm as of

July 31, 2008.

219   "A Sign of a Broken System," National Post (Canada), August 7, 2008.

220   "One in 5 Canadians Can't Find a Doctor: Survey," CTV, June 18, 2008, available at http://www.ctv.ca/servlet/ArticleNews/story/CTVNews/20080618/health_canadians_080618/20080618?hub=CTVNewsAt11 as of July 10, 2009.

221   See Nadeem Esmail and Michael A. Walker, "Waiting Your Turn: Hospital Waiting Lists in Canada," 17th Edition, Fraser Institute, October 15, 2007, available at http://www.fraserinstitute.org/commerce.web/product_files/WaitingYourTurn2007rev2.pdf as of July 22, 2009.

222   Tom Blackwell, "Ont. Doctor Uses Lotteries to Pare Down Patient List," National Post (Canada), August 5, 2008.

223   Ibid.

224   Dave Dale, "The Luck of the Draw," North Bay Nugget (Canada), July 22, 2008.

225   Tom Blackwell, "Ont. Doctor Uses Lotteries to Pare Down Patient List," National Post (Canada), August 5, 2008.

226   Ibid.

227   Ibid.

228   Ibid.

229   Dave Dale, "The Luck of the Draw," North Bay Nugget (Canada), July 22, 2008.

230   Tom Blackwell, "Ont. Doctor Uses Lotteries to Pare Down Patient List," National Post (Canada), August 5, 2008.

231   Pamela Fayerman, "MDs Won't Treat Disabled Child," Vancouver Sun (Canada), August 7, 2008, available at http://www.canada.com/vancouversun/health/story.html?id=2c996632-8dde-4ccd-bc90-15cda3afe796 as of July 22, 2009.

232   Ibid.

233   Ibid.

234   See MySpace page for Susan J. Watson, "About Me," available at http://www.myspace.com/463635427 as of June 11, 2009.

235   Susan Watson, Online Petition, "Please Help Carly," Care2.com, available at http://www.thepetitionsite.com/50/Please-Help-People-on-surgery-waitlists as of July 22, 2009.

236   Susan Watson, Internet comment to article by Pamela Fayerman, "New Children's Hospital Chief Quit U.S. Job amid Controversy," Vancouver Sun (Canada), June 25, 2008, available at http://www.canada.com/vancouversun/news/story.html?id=f245a0c8-5cc8-4de0-9150-044b23f4e20d as of July 22, 2009.

237   Susan Watson, Online Petition, "Please Help Carly," Care2.com, available at http://www.thepetitionsite.com/50/Please-Help-People-on-surgery-waitlists as of July 22, 2009.

238   Susan Watson and David Lamont, letter to the editor, "Young Lives Hang in the Balance," Vancouver Sun (Canada), May 31, 2008.

239   Ibid; Pamela Fayerman, "MDs Won't Treat Disabled Child," Vancouver Sun (Canada), August 7, 2008, available at http://www.canada.com/vancouversun/health/story.html?id=2c996632-8dde-4ccd-bc90-15cda3afe796 as of July 22, 2009.

240   Susan Watson, Online Petition, "Carly Arlene Lamont Denied Medical Care by Specialists and B.C. Children's Hospital," available at http://www.thepetitionsite.com/59/Please-Help-Carly-and-all-kids-on-these-outrageous-waitlists as of July 22, 2009.

241   Pamela Fayerman, "MDs Won't Treat Disabled Child," Vancouver Sun (Canada), August 7, 2008, available at http://www.canada.com/vancouversun/health/story.html?id=2c996632-8dde-4ccd-bc90-15cda3afe796 as of July 22, 2009.

242   Ibid.

243   Ibid.

244   Ibid.

245   Susan Watson, Online Petition, "Carly Arlene Lamont Denied Medical Care by Specialists and B.C. Children's Hospital," available at http://www.thepetitionsite.com/59/Please-Help-Carly-and-all-kids-on-these-outrageous-waitlists as of July 22, 2009.

246   Pamela Fayerman, "MDs Won't Treat Disabled Child," Vancouver Sun (Canada), August 7, 2008, available at http://www.canada.com/vancouversun/health/story.html?id=2c996632-8dde-4ccd-bc90-15cda3afe796 as of July 22, 2009.

247   Pamela Fayerman, "Nursing Shortage Hurting Children's Hospital," Vancouver Sun (Canada), May 23, 2008, available at http://www.canada.com/vancouversun/news/story.html?id=f35d9a68-9a33-4e31-868b-a06d11a76226 as of July 22, 2009.

248   Ibid.

249   For all source material and references, unless otherwise noted, see Stuart Laidlaw, "Woman 'Got My Life Back' after Surgery in India," Toronto Star (Canada), May 31, 2008, available at http://www.thestar.com/article/431891 as of July 22, 2009.

250   Mumtaz Pachisa, "Medical Tourism and Healthbase Help Canadian Bid Goodbye to Her Chronic Back Pain," Press Release, Healthbase, September 29, 2007, available at http://www.prlog.org/10032418-medical-tourism-and-healthbase-help-canadian-bid-goodbye-to-her-chronic-back-pain.html as of July 22, 2009.

251   Ibid.

252   Ibid.

AUSTRALIA

1   For all source material and references, unless otherwise noted, see Grant McArthur, "Patient's Patience Runs Out," Herald Sun (Australia), April 5, 2007, available at http://www.news.com.au/heraldsun/story/0,21985,21505526-2862,00.html as of July 22, 2009.

2   "The State of Our Public Hospitals, June 2006 Report: Are Patients Waiting Longer for Elective Surgery?," Department of Health and Ageing, Canberra, Australia, January 3, 2007.

3   For all source material and references, see "Granny Suffers 82 Hours of Agony," Sunday Times (Australia), May 19, 2007, available at http://www.news.com.au/perthnow/story/0,21598,21759824-2761,00.html as of July 8, 2009.

4   Paul Lampathakis, "Year's Wait for 30 Min Surgery," Sunday Times (Australia), April 1, 2007.

5   Paul Lampathakis, "Deaf Over Delay," Sunday Times (Australia), May 6, 2007.

6   Ibid; Paul Lampathakis, "Year's Wait for 30 Min Surgery," Sunday Times (Australia), April 1, 2007.

7   Paul Lampathakis, "Deaf Over Delay," Sunday Times (Australia), May 6, 2007.

8   Ibid.

9   Ibid.

10   Ibid; Paul Lampathakis, "Year's Wait for 30 Min Surgery," Sunday Times (Australia), April 1, 2007.

11   Paul Lampathakis, "Year's Wait for 30 Min Surgery," Sunday Times (Australia), April 1, 2007.

12   Hon. Kim Hames, "Surgery Cancelled Twice for 8-Year-Old," Media Statement, Office of the Leader of the Opposition, April 1, 2007.

13   Paul Lampathakis, "Deaf Over Delay," Sunday Times (Australia), May 6, 2007.

14   Paul Lampathakis, "Year's Wait for 30 Min Surgery," Sunday Times (Australia), April 1, 2007.

15   For all source material and references, unless otherwise noted, see Edith Bevin, "Horrendous Hospital Treatment," Daily Telegraph (Australia), April 11, 2008, available at http://www.news.com.au/dailytelegraph/story/0,22049,23518170-5006009,00.html as of July 22, 2009.

16   Adrienne Agg, "Miscarriage Leaves Couple in Anguish," Berwick and District Journal (Australia), April 7, 2008.

17   Ibid.

18   Troy Keams, "Rachel's Baby Agony," Pakenham Cardinia Leader (Australia), April 2, 2008.

19   According to the website of Casey Hospital, among its services offered are "a full range of imaging services including computed tomography, ultrasounds, nuclear medicine, cardiac stress testing and fluoroscopy; and has a 4 bed day ward for pre and post X-ray procedures." See "Casey Hospital Information for GPs," Casey Hospital, Berwick, Australia, available at http://www.southernhealth.org.au/gp/CaseyHospital.htm as of July 22, 2009.

20   Adrienne Agg, "Miscarriage Leaves Couple in Anguish," Berwick and District Journal (Australia), April 7, 2008.

21   Ibid.

22   Troy Keams, "Rachel's Baby Agony," Pakenham Cardinia Leader (Australia), April 2, 2008.

23   Adrienne Agg, "Miscarriage Leaves Couple in Anguish," Berwick and District Journal (Australia), April 7, 2008.

24   Ibid.

25   Ibid.

26   Troy Keams, "Rachel's Baby Agony," Pakenham Cardinia Leader (Australia), April 2, 2008.

27   Adrienne Agg, "Miscarriage Leaves Couple in Anguish," Berwick and District Journal (Australia), April 7, 2008.

28   Ibid.

29   Troy Keams, "Rachel's Baby Agony," Pakenham Cardinia Leader (Australia), April 2, 2008.

30   For all source material and references, unless otherwise noted, see Libby Bingham, "Pensioner's Life 'Is Hell' – 83-Year-Old Sits in Darkness during Four-Year Wait for Surgery," Advocate (Australia), April 19, 2008, available at http://nwtasmania.yourguide.com.au/news/local/news/general/pensioners-life-is-hell-83yearold-sits-in-darkness-during-fouryear-wait-for-surgery/199448.aspx as of July 22, 2009.

31   Ibid.

32   Libby Bingham, "Fast Response to Nellie's Plight – Cataract Operations Funded for Some, While Others." Advocate (Australia), April 24, 2008, available at http://nwtasmania.yourguide.com.au/news/local/news/general/fast-response-to-nellies-plight-cataract-operations-funded-for-some-while-others/199469.aspx as of July 22, 2009.

33   Ibid.

34   Kate Sikora, "RNS Denied Kathy Patsidis Forced into Toilet Birth," Daily Telegraph (Australia), May 7, 2008, available at http://www.news.com.au/dailytelegraph/story/0,22049,23657959-5006009,00.html as of July 22, 2009; "Baby Born in Sydney Hospital Toilet," Stuff (New Zealand), May 6, 2008, available at http://www.stuff.co.nz/4513172a12.html as of July 22, 2009.

35   "Report: Baby Born in Hospital Toilet," Australian (Australia), May 6, 2008.

36   "Baby Born in Sydney Hospital Toilet," Stuff (New Zealand), May 6, 2008, available at http://www.stuff.co.nz/4513172a12.html as of July 22, 2009.

37   Ibid.

38   "Woman Gives Birth in Sydney Hospital Toilet," New Zealand Herald (New Zealand), May 6, 2008.

39   "Baby Born in Sydney Hospital Toilet," Stuff (New Zealand), May 6, 2008, available at http://www.stuff.co.nz/4513172a12.html as of July 22, 2009.

40   "Woman Gives Birth in Sydney Hospital Toilet," New Zealand Herald (New Zealand), May 6, 2008.

41   Ibid.

42   "Baby Born in Sydney Hospital Toilet," Stuff (New Zealand), May 6, 2008, available at http://www.stuff.co.nz/4513172a12.html as of July 22, 2009.

43   Ibid; "Gran Slams Hospital over Toilet Baby," Sydney Morning Herald (Australia), May 7, 2008, available at http://news.smh.com.au/national/gran-slams-hospital-over-toilet-baby-20080507-2brj.html as of July 22, 2009.

44   "Second Woman Gives Birth in Sydney Hospital Toilet," Scopical (Australia), May 6, 2008, available at http://www.scopical.com.au/articles/News/5280/Second-woman-gives-birth-in-Sydney-hospital-toilet as of May 21, 2008.

45   "Baby Born in Sydney Hospital Toilet," Stuff (New Zealand), May 6, 2008, available at http://www.stuff.co.nz/4513172a12.html as of July 22, 2009.

46   Edwina Bartholomew, "Meager under Fire after Baby Born in Hospital Toilet," Live News (Australia), May 6, 2008.

47   "Woman Gives Birth in Sydney Hospital Toilet," New Zealand Herald (New Zealand), May 6, 2008.

48   "Baby Born in Sydney Hospital Toilet," Stuff (New Zealand), May 6, 2008, available at http://www.stuff.co.nz/4513172a12.html as of July 22, 2009.

49   Kate Sikora, "RNS Denies Claim: 'Baby Born in Toilet without Support,'" Daily Telegraph (Australia), May 6, 2008, available at http://www.news.com.au/dailytelegraph/story/0,22049,23653566-5006009,00.html as of July 22, 2009.

50   "Baby Born in Sydney Hospital Toilet," Stuff (New Zealand), May 6, 2008, available at http://www.stuff.co.nz/4513172a12.html as of July 22, 2009.

51   "Gran Slams Hospital over Toilet Baby," Sydney Morning Herald (Australia), May 7, 2008, available at http://news.smh.com.au/national/gran-slams-hospital-over-toilet-baby-20080507-2brj.html as of July 22, 2009.

52   For all source material and references, unless otherwise noted, see Sam Groves, "Three Year Old Waiting in Pain," Tenterfield Star (Australia), May 1, 2008, available at http://tenterfield.yourguide.com.au/news/local/news/general/three-year-old-waiting-in-pain/331508.aspx as of July 22, 2009.

53   Ibid; "Emergency Department for Life-Threatening Emergencies," Tenterfield Star (Australia), May 1, 2008, available at http://tenterfield.yourguide.com.au/news/local/news/general/emergency-department-for-lifethreatening-emergencies/510765.aspx as of July 22, 2009.

54   Lisa Finnerty and Sam Groves, "Hospital Disgrace – Three Kids Left to Wait in Two Weeks," Tenterfield Star (Australia), May 1, 2008, available at http://tenterfield.yourguide.com.au/news/local/news/general/hospital-disgrace-three-kids-left-to-wait-in-two-weeks/422096.aspx as of July 22, 2009.

55   Crystal Ja and Gabrielle Dunlevy, "Hospital Bed Shortage 'Could Happen Again,'" Brisbane Times (Australia), May 16, 2008, available at http://www.brisbanetimes.com.au/news/queensland/bed-shortage-could-happen-again/2008/05/15/1210765037125.html as of June 17, 2008.

56   Ben Dillaway, "Mum in Labour on Storeroom Floor," Gold Coast News (Australia), May 15, 2008, available at http://www.goldcoast.com.au/article/2008/05/15/11133_print_friendly.html as of June 17, 2008.

57   Crystal Ja and Gabrielle Dunlevy, "Hospital Bed Shortage 'Could Happen Again,'" Brisbane Times (Australia), May 16, 2008, available at http://www.brisbanetimes.com.au/news/queensland/bed-shortage-could-happen-again/2008/05/15/1210765037125.html as of June 17, 2008.

58   Ben Dillaway, "Mum in Labour on Storeroom Floor," Gold Coast News (Australia), May 15, 2008, available at http://www.goldcoast.com.au/article/2008/05/15/11133_print_friendly.html as of June 17, 2008.

59   Ibid.

60   Shannon Molloy, "Woman in Labour Forced to Lie on Hospital Floor," Brisbane Times (Australia), May 15, 2008, available at http://www.brisbanetimes.com.au/news/queensland/woman-in-labour-forced-to-lie-on-hospital-floor/2008/05/15/1210764997624.html as of June 17, 2008.

61   Ben Dillaway, "Mum in Labour on Storeroom Floor," Gold Coast News (Australia), May 15, 2008, available at http://www.goldcoast.com.au/article/2008/05/15/11133_print_friendly.html as of June 17, 2008.

62   Ibid.

63   Ibid.

64   Ibid.

65   Ibid.

66   Ibid.

67   "Birth Blunder Apology," Gold Coast (Australia), May 16, 2008, available at http://www.goldcoast.com.au/article/2008/05/16/11188_print_friendly.html as of June 17, 2008.

68   Crystal Ja and Gabrielle Dunlevy, "Hospital Bed Shortage 'Could Happen Again,'" Brisbane Times (Australia), May 16, 2008, available at http://www.brisbanetimes.com.au/news/queensland/bed-shortage-could-happen-again/2008/05/15/1210765037125.html as of June 17, 2008.

69   For all source material and references, unless otherwise noted, see Margo Ziotkowski, "Cancer Wait List Agonising," Cairns Post (Australia), May 31, 2008, available at http://www.cairns.com.au/article/2008/05/31/4260_local-news.html as of July 15, 2009.

70   "Qld Health Defends Cancer Patient Waits," Age (Australia), May 27, 2008, available at http://news.theage.com.au/national/qld-health-defends-cancer-patient-waits-20080527-2ij9.html as of July 15, 2009.

71   Alexandra Smith, "DIY Dentist Ends Four-Year Wait Agony," Sydney Morning Herald (Australia), June 25, 2008, available at http://www.smh.com.au/news/national/diy-dentist-ends-fouryear-wait-agony/2008/06/25/1214073313129.html as of July 15, 2009.

72   Jeffrey Miners, Radio Interview, "'I Was on Painkillers, I Couldn't Sleep': Mr Miners Explains," Radio 2GB (Australia), June 25, 2008.

73   Alexandra Smith, "DIY Dentist Ends Four-Year Wait Agony," Sydney Morning Herald (Australia), June 25, 2008, available at http://www.smh.com.au/news/national/diy-dentist-ends-fouryear-wait-agony/2008/06/25/1214073313129.html as of July 15, 2009.

74   Jeffrey Miners, Radio Interview, "'I Was on Painkillers, I Couldn't Sleep': Mr Miners Explains," Radio 2GB (Australia), June 25, 2008.

75   Alexandra Smith, "DIY Dentist Ends Four-Year Wait Agony," Sydney Morning Herald (Australia), June 25, 2008, available at http://www.smh.com.au/news/national/diy-dentist-ends-fouryear-wait-agony/2008/06/25/1214073313129.html as of July 15, 2009.

76   Jeffrey Miners, Radio Interview, "'I Was on Painkillers, I Couldn't Sleep': Mr Miners Explains," Radio 2GB (Australia), June 25, 2008.

77   Ibid.

78   Alexandra Smith, "DIY Dentist Ends Four-Year Wait Agony," Sydney Morning Herald (Australia), June 25, 2008, available at http://www.smh.com.au/news/national/diy-dentist-ends-fouryear-wait-agony/2008/06/25/1214073313129.html as of July 15, 2009.

79   Brett McKeehan, "Pensioner Jeffrey Miners Pulls Own Tooth in DIY Dentistry Scandal," Daily Telegraph (Australia), June 25, 2008, available at http://www.news.com.au/dailytelegraph/story/0,22049,23920386-5001021,00.html as of July 15, 2009.

80   "Man Pulls Own Tooth after 'Long Wait,'" Sydney Morning Herald (Australia), June 25, 2008, available at http://news.smh.com.au/national/man-pulls-own-tooth-after-long-wait-20080625-2wmu.html as of July 15, 2009.

81   Ibid.

82   Alexandra Smith, "DIY Dentist Ends Four-Year Wait Agony," Sydney Morning Herald (Australia), June 25, 2008, available at http://www.smh.com.au/news/national/diy-dentist-ends-fouryear-wait-agony/2008/06/25/1214073313129.html as of July 15, 2009.

83   Ibid.

84   "New South Wales," Encyclopedia Britannica, 2008, available at http://www.britannica.com/EBchecked/topic/412057/New-South-Wales as of July 15, 2009.

85   Alexandra Smith, "DIY Dentist Ends Four-Year Wait Agony," Sydney Morning Herald (Australia), June 25, 2008, available at http://www.smh.com.au/news/national/diy-dentist-ends-fouryear-wait-agony/2008/06/25/1214073313129.html as of July 15, 2009.

86   "Hospital Ignores Teen with Severed Fingers," Sunday Times (Australia), July 14, 2008, available at http://www.news.com.au/story/0,23599,24015491-1245,00.html as of July 10, 2009.

87   Ibid.

88   Ibid.

89   Joseph Catanzaro, "Anger at Long Hospital Wait after Losing Fingers," West Australian (Australia), July 14, 2008.

90   Ibid.

91   Ibid.

92   Ibid.

93   "Hospital Ignores Teen with Severed Fingers," Sunday Times (Australia), July 14, 2008, available at http://www.news.com.au/story/0,23599,24015491-1245,00.html as of July 10, 2009.

94   Ibid.

95   Ibid.

96   Joseph Catanzaro, "Anger at Long Hospital Wait after Losing Fingers," West Australian (Australia), July 14, 2008.

97   "Hospital Ignores Teen with Severed Fingers," Sunday Times (Australia), July 14, 2008, available at http://www.news.com.au/story/0,23599,24015491-1245,00.html as of July 10, 2009.

98   "About Us," Royal Perth Hospital, available at http://www.rph.wa.gov.au/about.html as of July 10, 2009.

99   "Hospital Ignores Teen with Severed Fingers," Sunday Times (Australia), July 14, 2008, available at http://www.news.com.au/story/0,23599,24015491-1245,00.html as of July 22, 2008.

100   Joseph Catanzaro, "Anger at Long Hospital Wait after Losing Fingers," West Australian (Australia), July 14, 2008.

101   Anthony Deceglie, "Teen Waited 28 Hours after Fingers Severed," Sunday Times (Australia), February 7, 2009, available at http://www.news.com.au/perthnow/story/0,21598,25021188-2761,00.html as of June 9, 2009.

102   "Four Hour Rule Program," Government of Western Australia Department of Health, available at http://www.health.wa.gov.au/fourhourrule/home/ as of June 9, 2009.

103   For all sources and references, unless otherwise noted, see Kathleen Donaghey, "Six-Year-Old Has Waited Two Years for Routine Surgery," Gold Coast Bulletin (Australia), August 9, 2008, available at http://www.goldcoast.com.au/article/2008/08/09/14749_print_friendly.html as of July 10, 2009.

104   "Quarterly Public Hospitals Performance Report," Queensland Health, June Quarter 2008, p. 9, available at http://

www.health.qld.gov.au/performance/docs/QPHPR_Jun_Qtr_08.pdf as of July 10, 2009.

105   Ibid., p. 6.

106   Ibid., p. 9.

107   For all source material and references, see Kamahl Cogdon, "Woman Faces 3-Year Surgery Wait," Herald Sun (Australia), July 2, 2007, available at http://www.news.com.au/heraldsun/story/0,21985,21999771-661,00.html as of June 23, 2009.

108   Grant McArthur, "400 Children Forced to Wait for Heart Surgery," Herald Sun (Australia), August 26, 2008, available at http://www.news.com.au/heraldsun/story/0,21985,24241300-661,00.html as of July 10, 2009.

109   Grant McArthur, "A Child Still Waits for Help as Operation Delayed," Herald Sun (Australia), August 29, 2008, available at http://www.news.com.au/heraldsun/story/0,21985,24258899-2862,00.html as of July 10, 2009.

110   Ibid.

111   Ibid.

112   Grant McArthur, "A Child Still Waits for Help as Operation Delayed," Herald Sun (Australia), August 29, 2008, available at http://www.news.com.au/heraldsun/story/0,21985,24258899-2862,00.html as of July 10, 2009.

113   Ibid.

114   Grant McArthur, "400 Children Forced to Wait for Heart Surgery," Herald Sun (Australia), August 26, 2008, available at http://www.news.com.au/heraldsun/story/0,21985,24241300-661,00.html as of July 10, 2009.

115   Ibid.

116   Ibid.

117   Grant McArthur, "Christmas Joy as a Cardiac Crisis is Solved," Herald Sun (Australia), December 15, 2008, available at http://www.news.com.au/heraldsun/story/0,,24799627-2862,00.html as of June 10, 2009.

118   For all source material and references, unless otherwise noted, see Alex Dickinson, "Bob Skinner's Long Hospital Wait with Mangled Hand," Courier-Mail (Australia), September 3, 2008, available at http://www.news.com.au/story/0,23599,24284959-2,00.html as of June 23, 2009.

119   See "About the Princess Alexandra Hospital Health Service District," Queensland Health, January 1, 2007, PAH Profile, available at http://www.health.qld.gov.au/pahospital/about_pa/default.asp as of June 23, 2009.

120   "Quarterly Public Hospitals Performance Report," Queensland Health, March Quarter 2009, p. 11, available at http://www.health.qld.gov.au/performance/docs/QPHPR_Mar_Qtr_09.pdf as of June 23, 2009.

121   Ibid., p. 11.

122   For all source material and references, unless otherwise noted, see Michelle Pountney, "Surgery Wait Hard to Swallow," Herald Sun (Australia), May 2, 2005.

123   Kate Jones, "Surgery Mum Set to Dine Out," Herald Sun (Australia), May 6, 2005.

124   Ibid.

125   For all source material and references, unless otherwise noted, see Angela Thompson, "Illawarra Woman Tells of Miscarriage Humiliation," Illawarra Mercury (Australia), January 13, 2009, available at http://www.illawarramercury.com.au/news/local/news/general/illawarra-woman-tells-of-miscarriage-humiliation/1405108.aspx as of February 13, 2009.

126   Clifford Hughes and William Walters, "Report of Inquiry into the Care of a Patient with Threatened Miscarriage at Royal North Shore Hospital on 25 September 2007," New South Wales Department of Health, October 26, 2007, available at http://www.health.nsw.gov.au/pubs/2007/pdf/inquiry_rnsh.pdf as of February 13, 2009.

SOUTH AFRICA

1   For all source material and references, unless otherwise noted, see Lynn Williams, "Mother's Harrowing Tale of Baby's Death," Herald (South Africa), March 26, 2008, available at http://www.theherald.co.za/herald/2008/03/26/news/n01_26032008.htm as of July 22, 2009, and Lynn Williams, "Money Won't Take Away Pain, Says Mom Who Sued Hospital," Weekend Post (South Africa), April 5, 2008, available at http://www.weekendpost.co.za/main/2008/04/05/news/nl10_05042008.htm as of July 22, 2009, and Lynn Williams, "Woman Who Lost Baby Wins Lawsuit," Herald (South Africa), March 31, 2008, available at http://www.theherald.co.za/herald/2008/03/31/news/n03_31032008.htm as of July 22, 2009.

2   Max Matavire, "Dora Nginza: 'The Situation Is A Crisis,'" Cape Times (South Africa), August 16, 2007, available at http://www.iol.co.za/index.php?set_id=1&click_id=13&art_id=vn20070816041643505C915130 as of July 22, 2009; "'One Nurse for 90 Patients,'" South African Press Association (South Africa), August 15, 2007, available at http://www.news24.com/News24/South_Africa/News/0,,2-7-1442_2165250,00.html as of July 22, 2009.

3   Max Matavire, "Dora Nginza: 'The Situation Is A Crisis,'" Cape Times (South Africa), August 16, 2007, available at http://www.iol.co.za/index.php?set_id=1&click_id=13&art_id=vn20070816041643505C915130 as of July 22, 2009.

4   Ibid.

5   For all sources and references, unless otherwise noted, see Antoinette Pienaar, "Hospital Blamed for Girl Dying," Beeld (South Africa), June 11, 2008, available at http://www.news24.com/News24/South_Africa/News/0,,2-7-1442_2338324,00.html as of July 22, 2009.

6   Thabisile Khoza, "Dead Baby's Records 'Missing,'" AfricanEye.org, July 7, 2008, available at http://www.news24.com/News24/South_Africa/News/0,,2-7-1442_2353218,00.html as of July 22, 2009.

7   For all source material and references, unless otherwise noted, see Daleen Naude, "Hospitals Unable to Deliver Baby," Citizen (South Africa), July 14, 2008, available at http://www.citizen.co.za/index/News/718809.page as of July 9, 2009, and Buks Viljoen, "'I'm Going to Lose My Child!',", Beeld (South Africa), July 16, 2008, available at http://www.news24.com/News24/South_Africa/News/0,,2-7-1442_2358120,00.html as of July 9, 2009.

8   For an audio recording, see "Dis Walglik!," Beeld (South Africa), October 29, 2008, available at http://jv.news24.com/Beeld/Video/0,,3-2082_2417923,00.html as of July 9, 2009.

9   For all source material and references, see Riot Hlatshwayo, "Nurses Probed after Mom Gives Birth in Toilet," Sowetan (South Africa), October 16, 2008, available at http://www.sowetan.co.za/News/Article.aspx?id=863975 as of July 22, 2009.

JAPAN

1   For all source materials and references, unless otherwise noted, see: "Man Dies after Being Refused Admission by 14 Hospitals," Associated Press, February 4, 2009, available at http://www.breitbart.com/article.php?id=D964IBAG0&show_article=1 as of July 23, 2009; Mari Yamaguchi, "Injured Man Dies after Rejection by 14 Hospitals," Associated Press, February 4, 2009; "Japanese ERs Turn Down Accident Victim," United Press International, February 4, 2009, available at http://www.upi.com/Top_News/2009/02/04/Japanese_ERs_turn_down_accident_victim/UPI-67461233758375/ as of July 23, 2009.

2   Chisaki Watanabe, "Survey Finds Japanese Hospitals Rejected 14,000 Emergency Patients in 2007," Associated Press, March 11, 2008, available at http://www.blnz.com/news/2008/03/11/Survey_finds_Japanese_hospitals_rejected_7098.html as of March 3, 2009.

3   "Pregnant Woman Refused by 18 Hospitals for Treatment, Later Dies," Japan Economic Newswire, October 17, 2006.

4   Hiroshi Osedo, "Tragedy as Pregnant Woman Turned away by 18 Hospitals," Courier Mail (Australia), October 21, 2006.

5   "Man Sues Town, Doc over Death of Pregnant Wife," Daily Yomiuri (Japan), May 24, 2007.

6   Ibid.

7   Hiroshi Osedo, "Tragedy as Pregnant Woman Turned away by 18 Hospitals," Courier Mail (Australia), October 21, 2006.

8   "Man Sues Town, Doc over Death of Pregnant Wife," Daily Yomiuri (Japan), May 24, 2007.

9   "Pregnant Woman Refused by 18 Hospitals for Treatment, Later Dies," Japan Economic Newswire, October 17, 2006.

10   "Man Sues Town, Doc over Death of Pregnant Wife," Daily Yomiuri (Japan), May 24, 2007.

11   "Comatose Woman in Labor Rejected by 18 Hospitals Dies," Japan Times (Japan), October 19, 2006, available at http://search.japantimes.co.jp/cgi-bin/nn20061019a3.html as of April 20, 2009.

12   Hiroshi Osedo, "Tragedy as Pregnant Woman Turned away by 18 Hospitals," Courier Mail (Australia), October 21, 2006.

13   Ibid.

14   "Comatose Woman in Labor Rejected by 18 Hospitals Dies," Japan Times (Japan), October 19, 2006, available at http://search.japantimes.co.jp/cgi-bin/nn20061019a3.html as of April 20, 2009.

15   "Man Sues Town, Doc over Death of Pregnant Wife," Daily Yomiuri (Japan), May 24, 2007.

16   Hiroshi Osedo, "Tragedy as Pregnant Woman Turned away by 18 Hospitals," Courier Mail (Australia), October 21, 2006.

RUSSIA

1   For all source material and references, unless otherwise noted, see LiveJournal User Lassi, "Need Advice, Guys… Saint-Petersburg," LiveJournal, October 10, 2008, available at http://users.livejournal.com/lassi_/7545.html as of January 23, 2009; document translated for authors by Victoria Strokova; and LiveJournal User Nisovsky, "About Self-Respect," LiveJournal, October 19, 2008, available at http://nisovsky.livejournal.com/143725.html as of January 23, 2009; document translated for authors by Victoria Strokova.

SWEDEN

1   Waldemar Ingdahl, "His Hip, Hooray!" TSCDaily, June 4, 2004, available at http://www.tcsdaily.com/article.aspx?id=060404D as of January 5, 2009.

2   Ibid.

3   "Equal-Opportunity Suffering," Editorial, Chattanooga Times Free Press, May 31, 2004.

4   Waldemar Ingdahl, "His Hip, Hooray!" TSCDaily, June 4, 2004, available at http://www.tcsdaily.com/article.aspx?id=060404D as of January 5, 2009.

5   "Swedish PM to Wait in Line for Hip Operation," Reuters, May 25, 2004, available at http://www.freerepublic.com/focus/f-news/1142285/posts as of January 5, 2009.

6   Waldemar Ingdahl, "His Hip, Hooray!" TSCDaily, June 4, 2004, available at http://www.tcsdaily.com/article.aspx?id=060404D as of January 5, 2009.

7   Ibid.

8   "Ministers Humble and Hip," Local (Sweden), June 4, 2004, available at http://www.thelocal.se/208/20040604/ as of June 12, 2009.

9   "Swedish PM to Wait in Line for Hip Operation," Reuters, May 25, 2004, available at http://www.freerepublic.com/focus/f-news/1142285/posts as of January 5, 2009.

10   Pia Maria Jonsson, et al., "Health Care: Status Report 2003," The National Board of Health and Welfare, 2003, p. 13, available at http://www.socialstyrelsen.se/NR/rdonlyres/1DA644DE-5036-43C5-A186-3DC31171F021/2519/summary.pdf as of January 5, 2009.

11   Waldemar Ingdahl, e-mail to Ryan Balis, December 20, 2008.

12   David Hogberg, Ph.D., "Sweden's Single-Payer Health System Provides a Warning to Other Nations," National Policy Analysis #555, May 2007, available online at http://www.nationalcenter.org/NPA555_Sweden_Health_Care.html.

13   Sven R. Larson, Ph.D., "Lessons from Sweden's Universal Health System:

Tales from the Health-care Crypt," Journal of American Physicians and Surgeons, Volume 13, Number 1, Spring 2008, available online at http://www.jpands.org/vol13no1/larson.pdf as of July 21, 2009.

14   Ibid.

15   "Mammography at Risk in Sweden, Says Cancerfonden," press release, International Union Against Cancer, October 3, 2007, available online at http://www.uicc.org/index.php?option=com_content&task=view&id=16003&Itemid=63 as of July 16, 2009.

NEW ZEALAND

1   Unless otherwise noted, for all source material and references, see Martin Johnston, "Urgent Test for Cancer Offered Two Years Late," New Zealand Herald (NZ), July 23, 2007, available at http://www.nzherald.co.nz/section/1/story.cfm?c_id=1&objectid=10453220&pnum=0 as of July 10, 2009.

2   "Otago Study Identifies Key Factors in Reducing Colorectal Cancer," Dunedin School of Medicine, University of Otago, Dunedin, NZ, August 26, 2005, available at http://www.otago.ac.nz/news/news/2005/26-08-05_press_release.html as of July 10, 2009.

3   See also Cancer Research Charitable Trust, available at http://www.cancerresearch.org.au/nz.html as of July 10, 2009.

4   For all source material and references, see Rob Kerr, "Mother Angry at Hospital's Lack of Caring," The Timaru Herald (Stuff.co.nz) (New Zealand), November 11, 2008, available at http://www.stuff.co.nz/4757572a20475.html as of June 24, 2009.

5   For all source material and references, unless otherwise noted, see Katie Wylie, "Woman Left with Unfinished Surgery," The Press (Stuff.co.nz), September 30, 2008.

6   "Endometriosis," MedlinePlus [Online], U.S. National Library of Medicine and National Institutes of Health, September 14, 2008, available at http://www.nlm.nih.gov/medlineplus/endometriosis.html as of July 15, 2009.

7   For all source material and references, see 3News Television Interview on Michael Wigmore, "Hospital Tells Man Suffering Stroke to Wait in Lazy-Boy Chair," 3News (New Zealand), September 3, 2008, video available at http://www.3news.co.nz/Video/National/tabid/309/articleID/69880/cat/17/Default.aspx#video as of July 8, 2009, and "Hospital Tells Man Suffering Stroke to Wait in Lazy-Boy Chair," 3News (New Zealand), September 3, 2008, available at http://www.3news.co.nz/National/Story/tabid/423/articleID/69880/cat/17/Default.aspx as of July 8, 2009.